MONOPOLY BUREAU
GOVERNMENT OF FORMOSA

Investigation
of the
Shô-Gyū and Yu-Ju Oils
Produced in Formosa

By

Kazuo Nagai

British Library Cataloguing-in-Publication Data
A catalogue record for this book is available from the
British Library

Essential Oils

Essential oils are also known as volatile oils, ethereal oils, aetherolea, or simply as the 'oil of' the plant from which they are extracted, such as the oil of clove. An oil is 'essential' in the sense that it contains the characteristic fragrance of the plant that it is taken from. Essential oils do not form a distinctive category for any medicinal, pharmacological, or culinary purpose - and they are not essential for health, although they have been used medicinally in history. Although some are suspicious or dismissive towards the use of essential oils in healthcare or pharmacology, essential oils retain considerable popular use, partly in fringe medicine and partly in popular remedies. Therefore it is difficult to obtain reliable references concerning their pharmacological merits.

Medicinal applications proposed by those who sell or use medical oils range from skin treatments to remedies from cancer - and are generally based on historical efficacy. Having said this, some essential oils such as those of juniper and agathosma are valued for their diuretic effects. Other oils, such as clove oil or eugenol were popular for many hundreds of years in dentistry and as antiseptics and local anaesthetics. However as the use of essential oils has declined in evidence based medicine, older text-books are frequently our only sources for information! Modern works are less inclined to generalise; rather than referring to 'essential oils' as a class at all, they prefer to discuss specific compounds, such as methyl salicylate, rather than 'oil of wintergreen.'

Nevertheless, interest in essential oils has considerably revived in recent decades, with the popularity of aromatherapy, alternative health stores and massage. Generally, the oils are volatized or diluted with a carrier oil to be used in massage, or diffused in the air by a nebulizer, heated over a candle flame, or burned as incense. Their usage goes way back, and the earliest recorded mention of such methods used to produce essential oils was made by Ibn al-Baitar (1188-1248), an Andalusian physician, pharmacist and chemist. Different oils were claimed to have differing properties; some to have an uplifting and energizing effect on the mind such as grapefruit and jasmine, whilst others such as rose lavender have a reputation as de-stressing and relaxing - and also, usefully, as an insect repellent.

The oils themselves are usually extracted by 'distillation', often by using steam -but some other processes include 'expression' or 'solvent extraction'. Distillation involves raw plant material (be that flowers, leaves, wood, bark, roots, seeds or peel) put into an alembic (distillation apparatus) over water. As the water is heated, the steam passes through the plant material, vaporizing the volatile compounds. The vapours flow through a coil, where they condense back to liquid, which is then collected in the receiving vessel. 'Expression' differs in that it usually merely uses a mechanical or cold press to extract the oil. Most citrus peel oils are made in this way, and due to the relatively large quantities of oil in citrus peel and low cost to grow and harvest the raw materials, citrus-fruit oils are cheaper than most other essential oils. 'Solvent extraction' is perhaps the most difficult of the three methods, and is generally used for flowers, which contain too little volatile oil to undergo expression. Instead, a solvent such as hexane or supercritical carbon dioxide is used to extract the oils.

These techniques have allowed essential oils to be used in all manner of products; from perfumes to cosmetics, soaps - and as flavourings for food and drinks as well as adding scent to incense and household cleaning products. The science, history and folkloric tradition of essential oils is incredibly fascinating - and a still much debated area. We hope the reader is inspired by this book to find out more.

PREFACE.

The Island of Formosa is situated, as is well known, in the southern extremity of our Empire, with a portion extending into the tropics. The climate is, therefore, moderately warm and humid throughout the year, and the growth and exuberance of vegetation in widely varied forms, is truly remarkable. The traveller, as he passes through the remote mountainous region or savage districts, is struck at once by the majestic and impressive features of the densely wooded forest; of the huge primeval trees twisting and interlocking their branches; and of the beauty and splendour of the tropical vegetation, which is strongly suggestive of an atmosphere of eternal verdure and perpetual summer. These marvellous features, so peculiar and distinctive, sufficiently illustrate the vast natural resources of forest products, of which camphor, dominating the world in the amount of its production, is the typical representative.

The parent-tree, *Cinnamomum Camphora*, from which our camphor is produced, is found abundantly in every prefecture, and not only supplies annually an enormous quantity of camphor to the world's market, but is capable of producing it to a still larger amount, should occasion demand; therefore, it is not exaggerating to say that this resource is almost unlimited.

As the result of investigations in connection with the camphor-producing industry, there is a firm conviction that the forests of Formosa are extremely rich in various species of perennial trees, closely allied to the camphor tree. Consequently, it is not unreasonable to assume that the encouragement and efforts directed towards the manufacture of oils from these woods will undoubtedly open a vast field for the expansion of our productive industries.

The *Shiu-Shô* tree, which thrives in the camphor regions, in association with the camphor tree, but which was formerly considered as of no value, has recently been shown by scientific investigations to be capable of playing a prominent part as material for the production of camphor or linalool, furnishing a fair example of possible development. Stimulated by the initial success, we have, in co-operation with others concerned in the industry, undertaken a gradual and systematic investigation of sources for essential oils, and the work has now progressed to such a stage as to be able to announce that we are about to reach a successful conclusion, in more than one way, in compensation for our laborious undertakings.

The object of this work is to publish the results of studies of several essential oils produced from trees, which, ranking next to the *Shiu-Shô* tree, are found abundantly in the primeval forests of Formosa ; and also to prove that the foregoing opinions regarding the prospects of the essential oil industry are not mere speculations.

Part I embraces a consideration covering investigations of a newly discovered essential oil obtained from a tree called " *Shô-Gyū*," closely resembling the camphor tree in external appearance. From an investigation of the *Shô-Gyū* tree in several prefectures, there seems to be a strong possibility of its flourishing along the central mountain range, forming an isolated belt parallel to the camphor region, and spreading over an extensive area. Hitherto, the tree had been wholly neglected by our industrial promoters, and no attention had been directed towards the utilization and development of this valuable natural resource, except an occasional indiscriminate cutting of timber. An experimental manufacture of oil from it, followed by the investigation of its chemical properties, was accordingly carried out sometime ago by the order and under the supervision of this Bureau. Subsequent results showed that *Shô-Gyū* oil, together with *Shiu* oil, occupies a most favourable position among rival essential oils, justifying itself to be classed among the special products of Formosa.

It is, therefore, with profound satisfaction, as well as a sense of justice, that we submit to the public a concise account of our studies.

Problems relating to the chemical investigation of an essential oil produced from a species of the southern camphor tree, commonly called " *Yu-Ju* ", are also dealt with. One of the distinctive features of the Formosan camphor tree, as the manufacturers of camphor are well aware, is the variation in the amount of camphor contained, according to the latitude. In the northern region, the stearoptene contained reaches the maximum quantity, and as one goes south it gradually diminishes, until its complete absence is occassionally noted. The oil thus failing to yield camphor through the usual process of manufacture is called " *Yu-Ju* Oil "; and its characteristic features having been determined as differing from the genuine camphor oil, it is discussed in Part II of these investigations.

Inasmuch as the special forest products of Formosa, other than camphor and *Shiu* oils, such as the above-mentioned *Shô-Gyū* and *Yu-Ju* oils, with a promise of producing them in considerable quantity, are being successively discovered and brought under our notice, the island forests undisputedly deserve to enjoy the reputation of possessing a valuable source of wealth for the production of essential oils.

Furthermore, there is every indication that upon the establishment of better means of communication with the savage districts, and along with their development, numerous valuable materials worthy of investigation, with a view to promoting our essential oil industry, may be obtained.

K. NAGAI.

February, 1913.

MAP OF FORMOSA
—SHOWING THE DISTRIBUTION OF SHÔ-GYŪ AND YU-JU TREES—

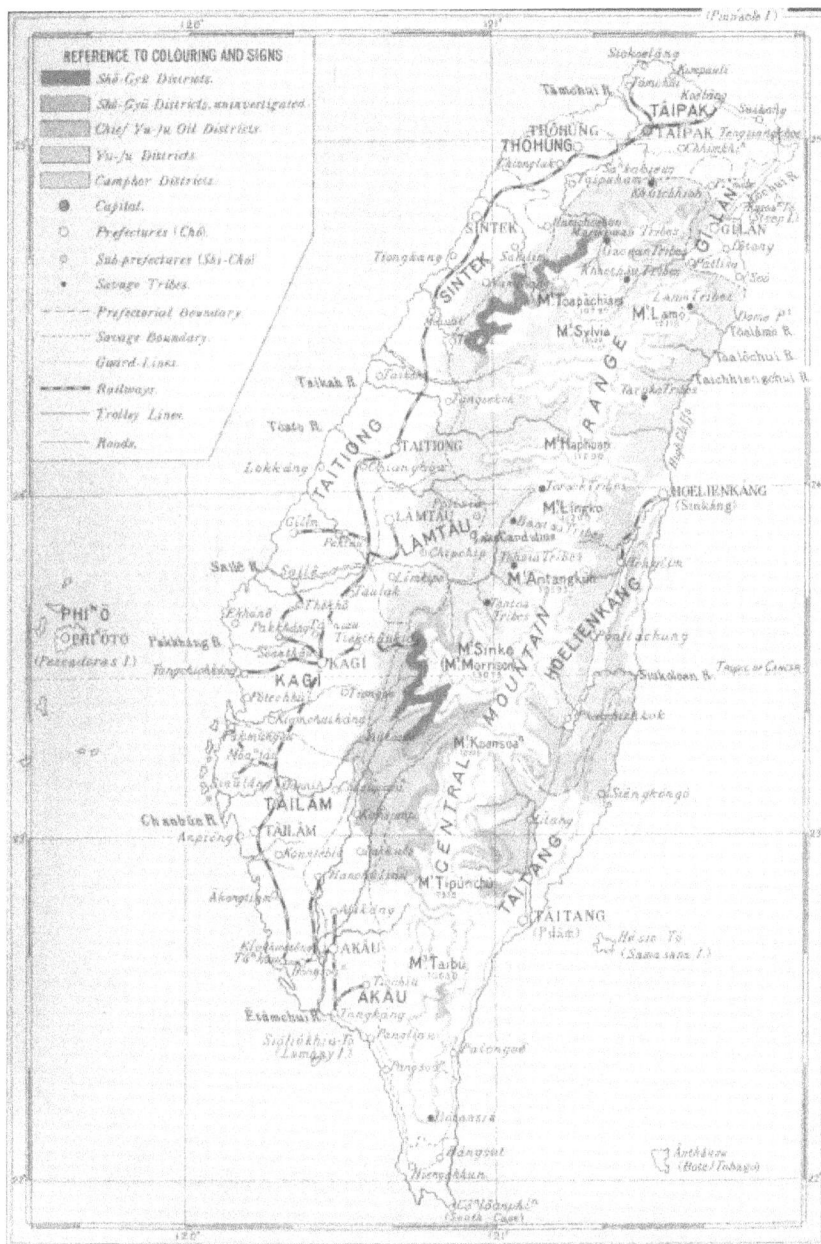

(Pinnacle I.)

REFERENCE TO COLOURING AND SIGNS

- Shô-Gyū Districts.
- Shô-Gyū Districts, uninvestigated.
- Chief Yu-Ju Oil Districts.
- Yu-Ju Districts.
- Camphor Districts.
- ● Capital.
- ○ Prefectures (Chō).
- ○ Sub-prefectures (Shi-Chō).
- • Savage Tribes.
- ---- Prefectorial Boundary.
- —— Savage Boundary.
- —— Guard-Lines.
- ■■■ Railways.
- —— Trolley Lines.
- —— Roads.

Siokoelang
Kampanli
Tamchui R.
Koehing
Suskoeng
TAIPAK
THOHUNG
THOHUNG
TAIPAK
Tenguangchoe
Ohimki
Khiichioh
GILAN
SINTEK
Manchochon
Maruseus Tribes
GILAN
Detony
Sei
Tiongkang
SINTEK
Sabsia
Khaichiu Tribes
Tatting
M. Toapachian
Lamn Tribes
M. Lamo
Mono P.
M. Sylvia
Toalhmo R.
Taalochui R.
Taikah R.
Taichhiongchui R.
TAITIONG
Toato R.
M. Haphuan
Lokkáng
TAITIONG
Chunghoa
Jarock Tribes
HOELIENKANG
(Sinkáng)
M. Lingco
LAMTAU
Baarai Tribes
LAMTAU
Camdulins
Theia Tri-Bes
M. Antangkuh
Sale
Limkos
Tantoa
Tribes
M. Sinko
(M. Morrison)
KAGI
HOELIENKANG
PHI'Ō
PEH'OTO
Pakhuang B.
(Pescadores I.)
KAGI
M. Koamsoa
Siukohoan R.
Tropic of Cancer
TAILAM
Siénkongó
Lisng
Chsabbia R.
TAILAM
TAITANG
Anpieng
M. Tipunchu
CENTRAL MOUNTAIN
Akongtins
TAITANG
(Pdam)
AKAU
Hesie To
(Sama sana I.)
M. Taibu
AKAU
Evamchui R.
Tongkang
Panolias
Patongoé
Pingso
Bangsut
Anthonu
Hengchhun
(Hote I Tobago)
S. Bangkih
(South Cape)

Scale 1:2.000.000   Height in Feet
Japanese Ri   English Miles

MAP OF SHIN-CHIKU PREFECTURE
— SHOWING THE GROWING DISTRICTS OF SHÔ-GYŪ TREES —

REFERENCE TO COLOURING AND SIGNS

▨ Shô-Gyū Districts.	∗ Tribes of Aborigines.
▨ Shô-Gyū Districts, uninvestigated.	⊙ Savage Police Stations. / Guards' Superintendent Stations.
☐ Camphor Districts.	----- Boundary of Prefecture.
⊚ Seat of Prefecture (Chô).	------ Boundary of Savage District.
◎ Seats of Sub-prefectures (Shi-Chô).	
○ Native (Formosan) Villages.	·········· Roads.

----- Guard Lines.
--ᴵ-- Railways.
----- Trolley Lines.

Scale 1:500.000
Japanese Ri

Height in Feet
English Miles

MAP OF KA-GI PREFECTURE

— SHOWING THE GROWING DISTRICTS OF SHÔ-GYŪ AND YU-JU TREES —

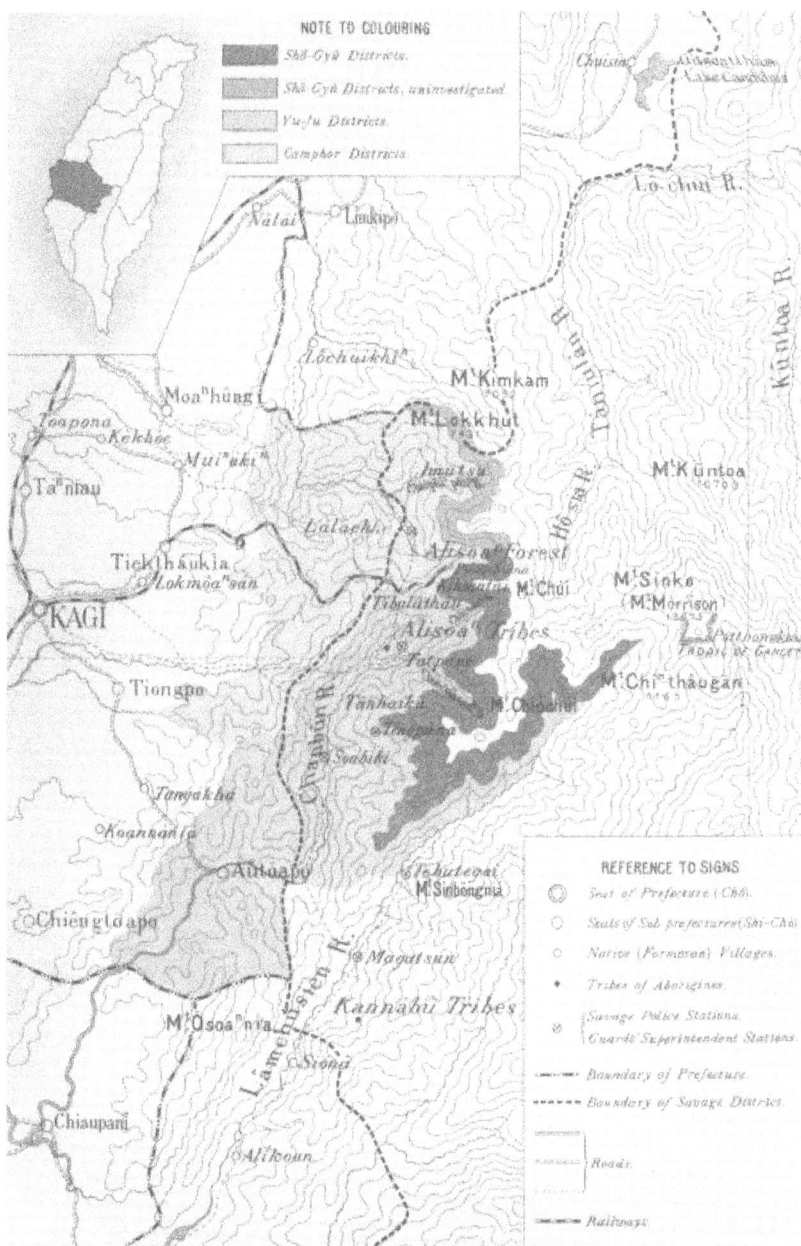

NOTE TO COLOURING

Shô-Gyû Districts.

Shô-Gyû Districts, uninvestigated

Yu-Ju Districts.

Camphor Districts

Chuisia

Lo-chut R.

Küntoa R.

Nàlai　Limkpà

A.bchuikhi

Moaⁿhûng

Toopona
Kelchoc

Muiⁿuki

M.Kimkam

M.Lokkhut

Imutou

Taⁿniau

Lalachi

Alisoa Forest

M.Chúi

M.Küntoa

Tickhāukia
Lokmōaⁿsan

KAGI

Tibulathau

Alisoa Tribes

Tatpou

M.Sinko
(M.Morrison)

Tiongpo

Tanhaika
Tongpou

Soabiki

M.Osochui

M.Chiⁿthaugan

Tanyakha

Koankania

Autoapo

Tchutegai
M.Sinhengnia

Chiéugtoapo

Magutsun

Kannahū Tribes

M.Osoaⁿnia

Stona

Chiaupani

Aliboun

REFERENCE TO SIGNS

Seat of Prefecture (Chô).

Seats of Sub-prefectures (Shi-Chô)

Native (Formosan) Villages.

Tribes of Aborigines.

Savage Police Stations.
Guards' Superintendent Stations.

Boundary of Prefecture

Boundary of Savage District.

Roads.

Railways.

Scale 1:500,000

Japanese　Ri

Height in Feet

English　Miles

MAP OF A-KŌ PREFECTURE
— SHOWING THE GROWING DISTRICTS OF SHŌ-GYŪ AND YU-JU TREES —

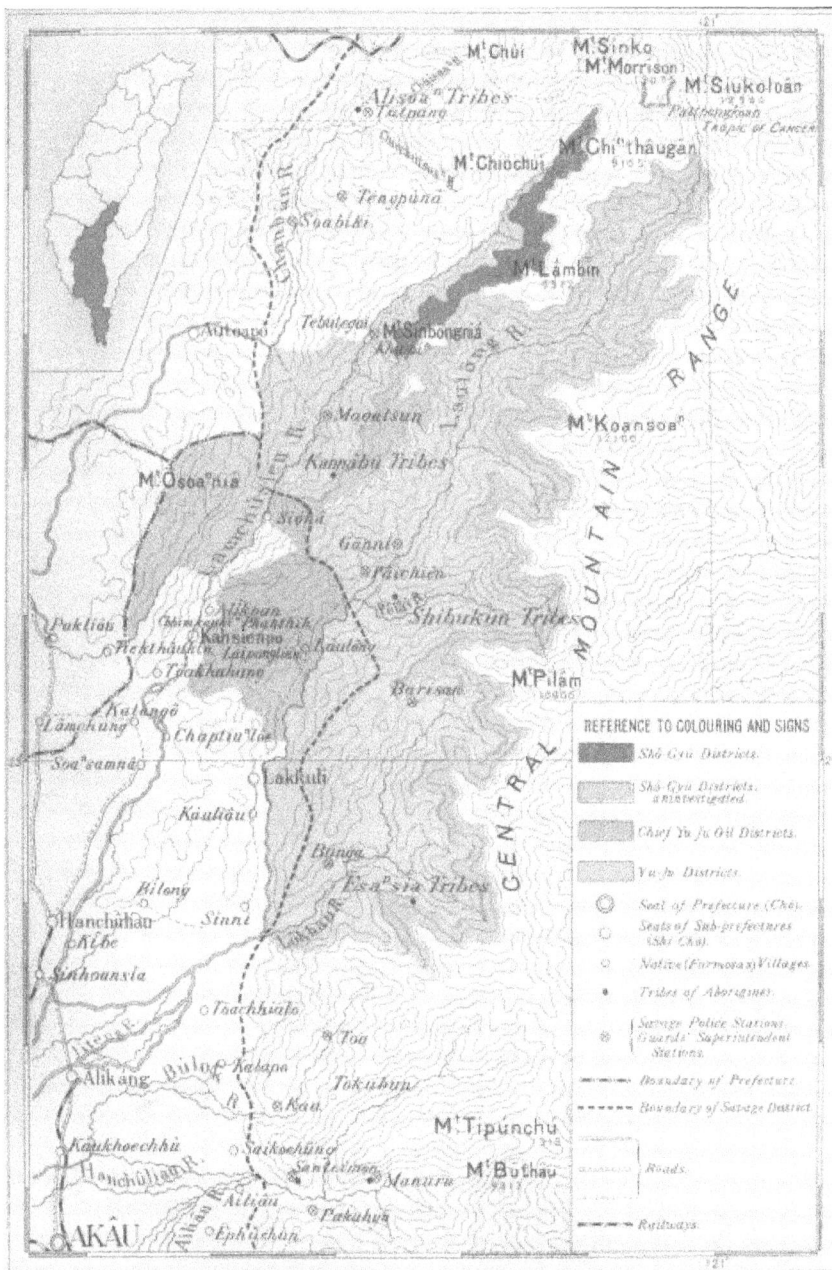

M. Chui
M. Sinko
(M. Morrison)
M. Siukoloan
Absoa Tribes
Tatpang
Paksiaukoan
Tropic of Cancer
M. Chi'thaugan
M. Chiochui
Tenopuna
Soabiki
Chianban R.
M. Lambin
Autoapo
Tebulegoi
M. Sinbongna
Atako
Laolong R.
Maoatsun
M. Koansoa
Kanabu Tribes
M. Osoa'nia
Sigha
Ganni
Paichien
Shibukun Tribes
Akhan Phasalik
Paklian
Kahsiehpo
Chimpoa
Tekthaukou
Laipangloa
Kauloro
Toakkahuno
M. Pilam
Barisan
Katango
Lamohung
Chaptiu'loa
Soa'samna
Lakkuli
Kauliau
Binga
Bilong
Esa'sia Tribes
Hanchihau
Aibe
Sinni
Lakkau
Sinhounsia
Toachhialo
Toa
CENTRAL MOUNTAIN RANGE
Alikang
Bulo
Katapa
Tokuhun
Li
Kao
M. Tipunchu
Kaukhoechhu
Saikoehun
Hanchulian R.
Santewan
Manuru
M. Buthau
Aitau
Takuhun
AKAU
Ephuchun

REFERENCE TO COLOURING AND SIGNS

Shō-Gyu Districts.

Shō-Gyu Districts, uninvestigated.

Chief Yu-Ju Oil Districts.

Yu-Ju Districts.

○ Seat of Prefecture (Cho).

○ Seats of Sub-prefectures (Shi Cho).

○ Native (Formosan) Villages.

• Tribes of Aborigines.

⊛ Savage Police Stations (Guards' Superintendent Stations.)

Boundary of Prefecture

Boundary of Savage District

Roads.

Railways.

Scale 1:500,000   Height in Feet
Japanese   Ri   English   Miles

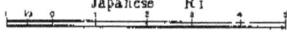

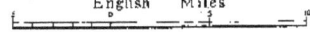

PART I

Investigation of the Essential Oil
of *Shô-Gyū*

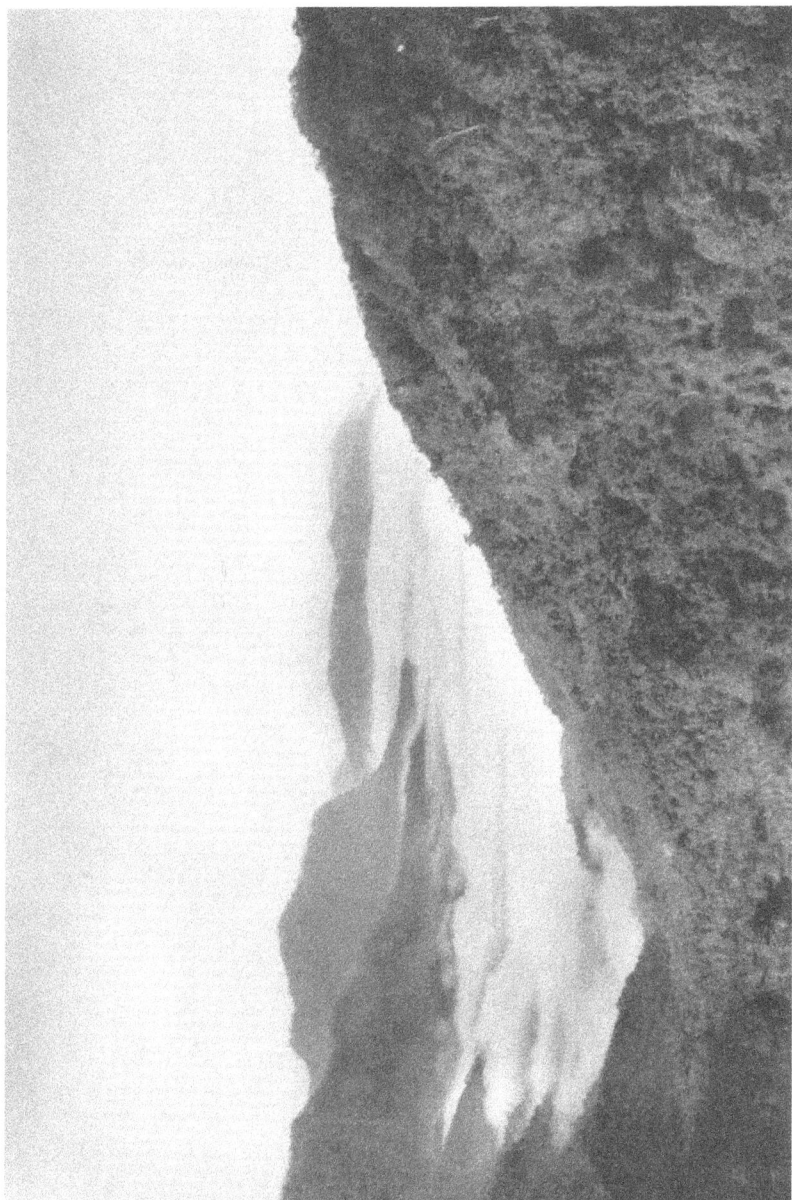

Mountain view from *Punkiko* on the *Arisan* road.

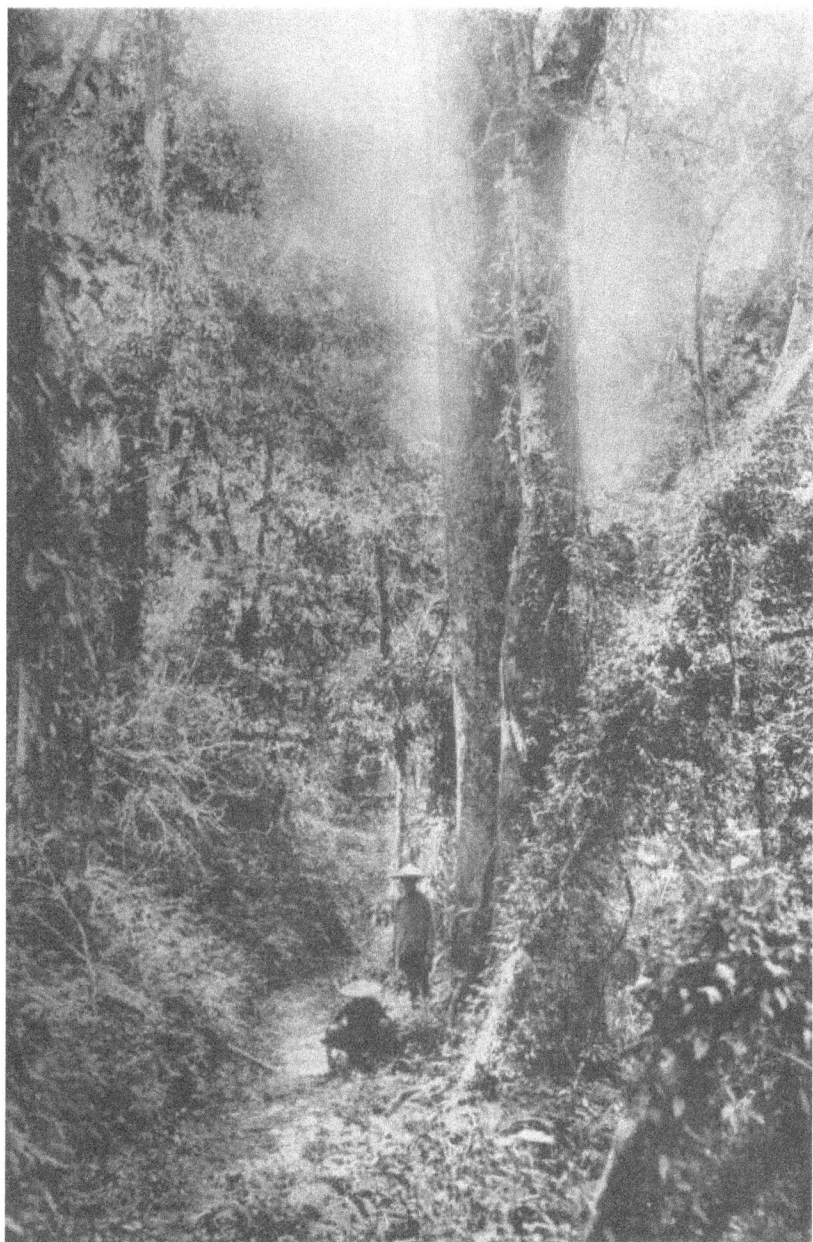

Shō-Gyŭ trees on *Kikwandai* hill along the old *Arisan* road.

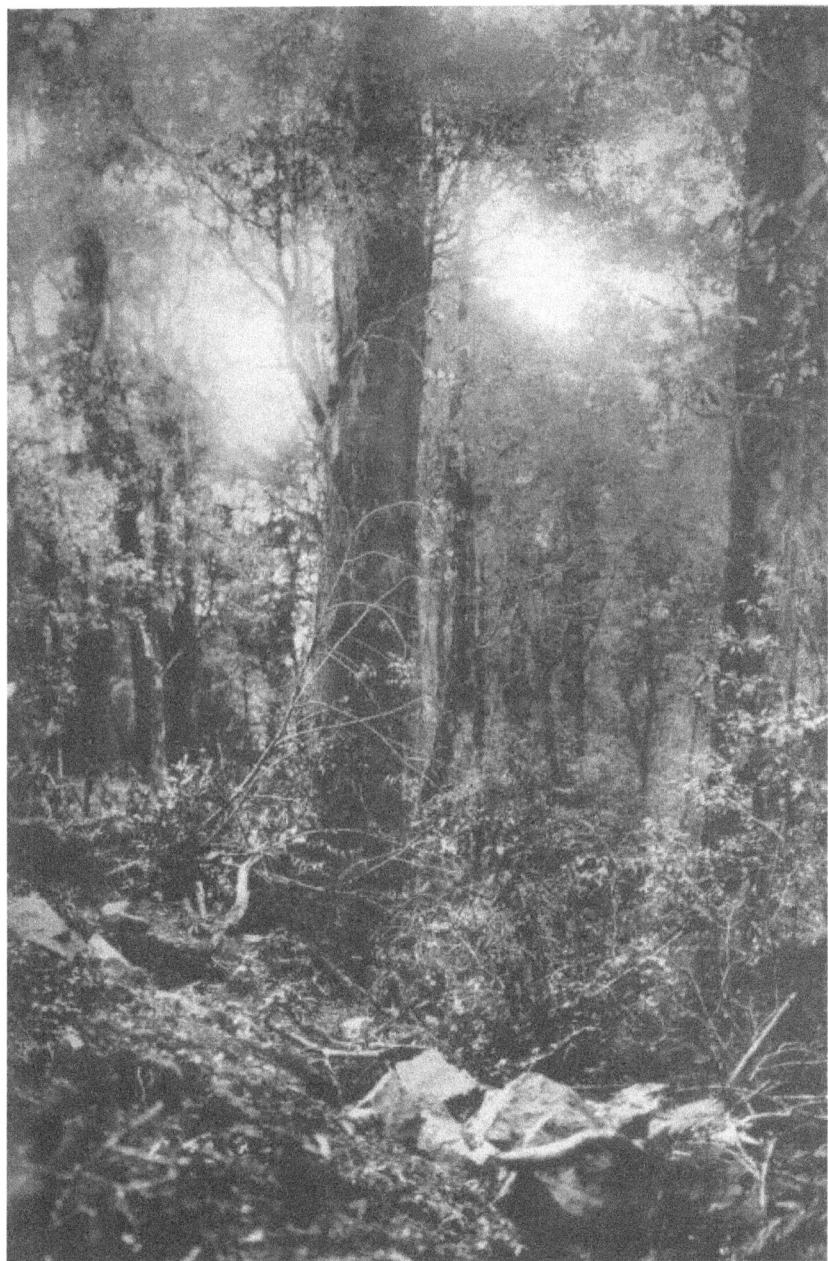

Shō-Gyū trees in *Nimandaira.*

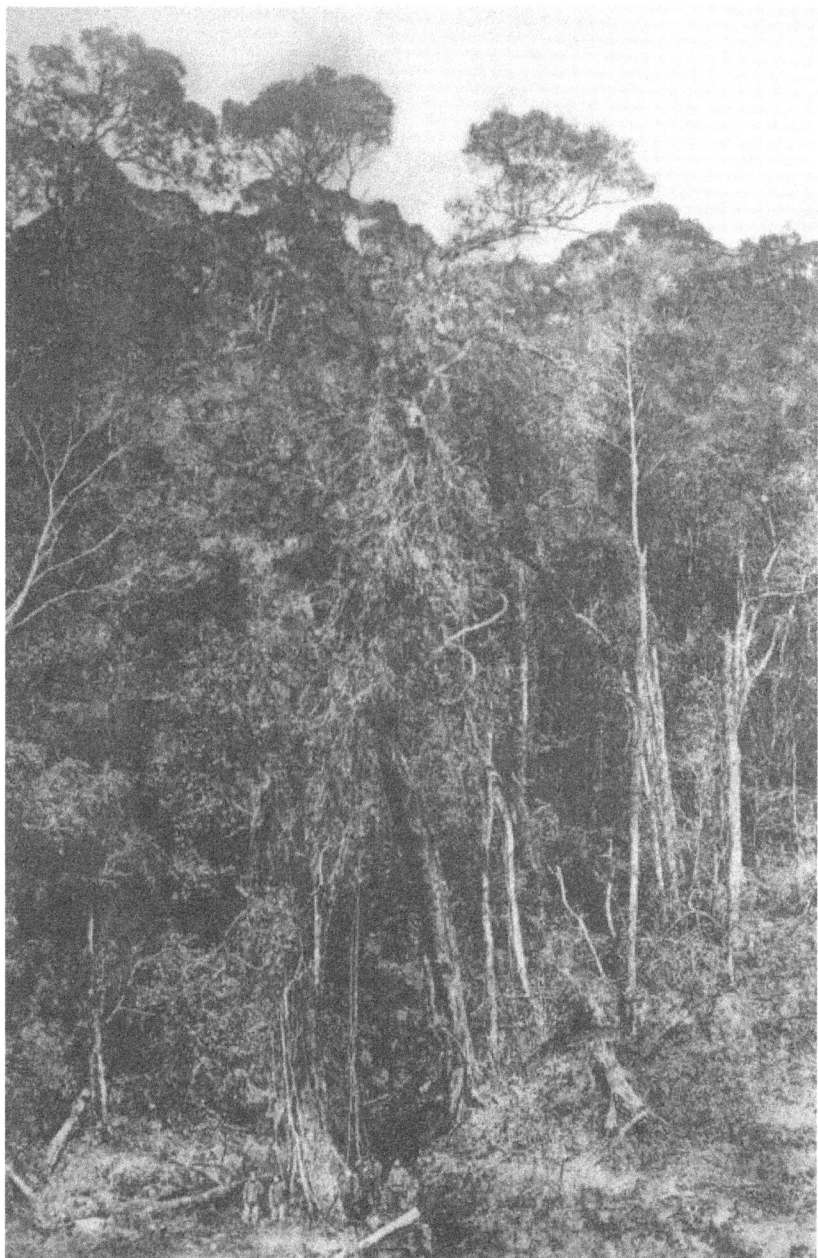

Shô-Gyū forest in *Heishana*.

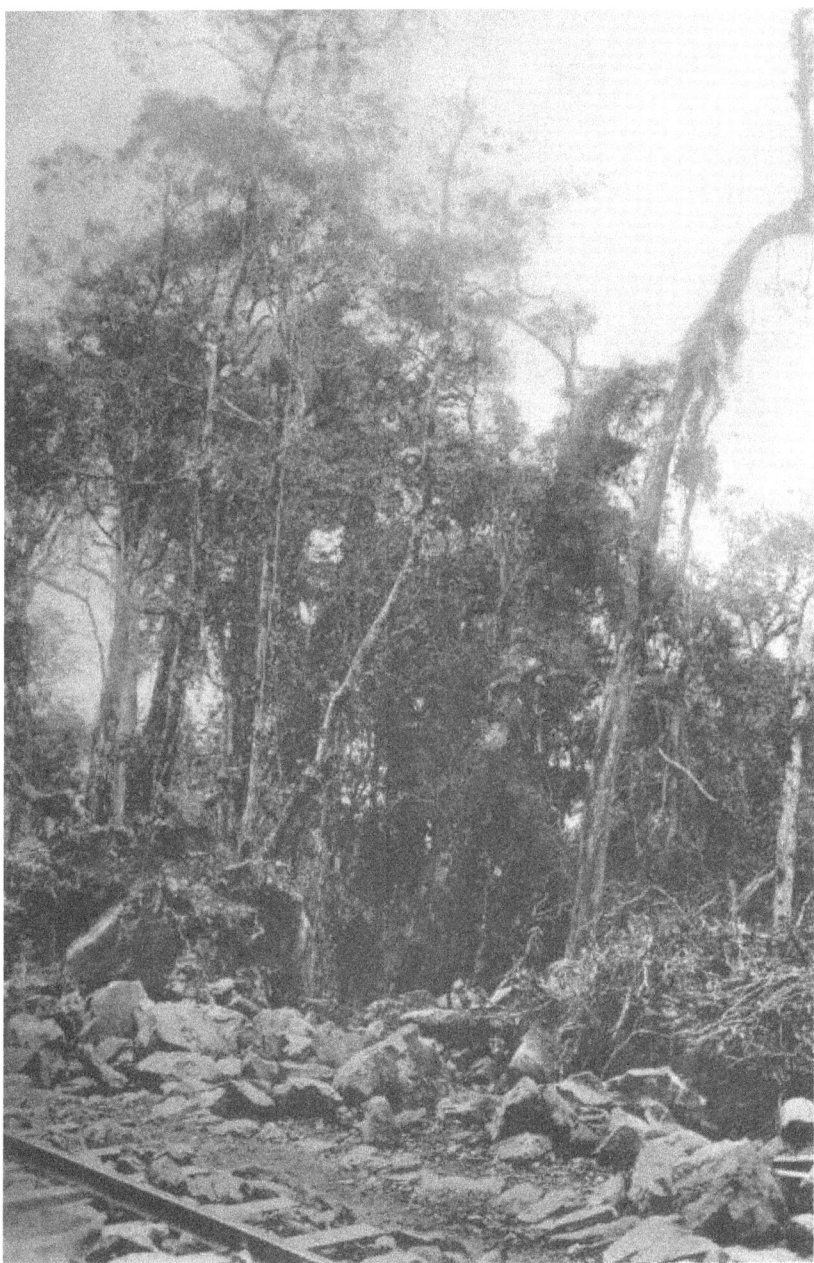

Shō-Gyū forest in vicinity of *Heishana.*

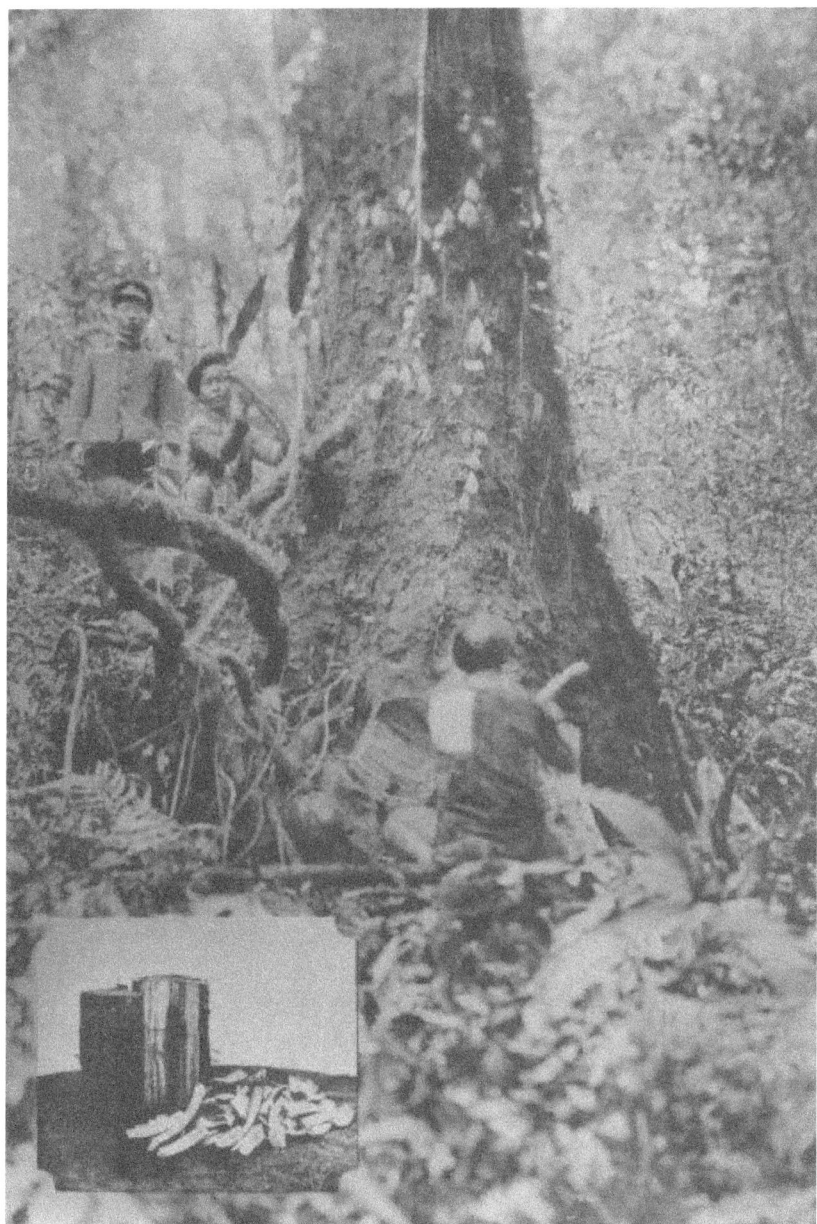

Chopping the trunk of *Shô-Gyū*.

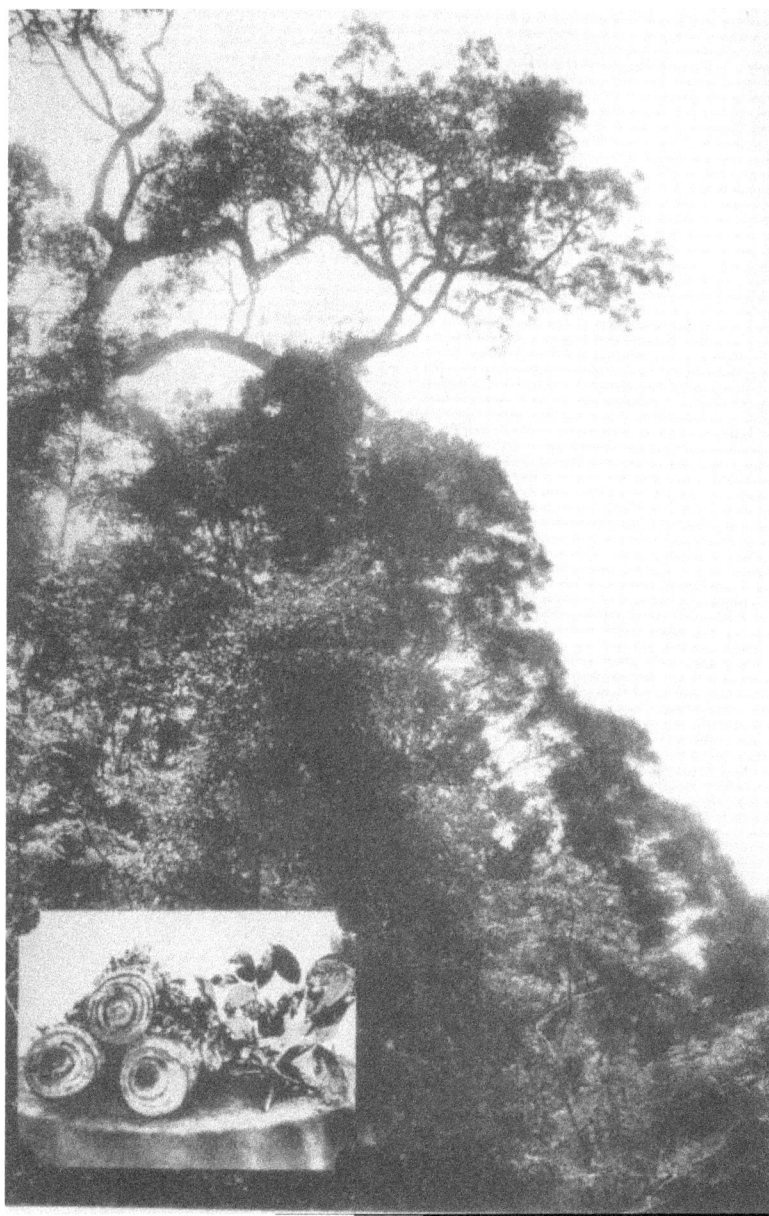

Branches and twigs of *Shô-Gyū*.

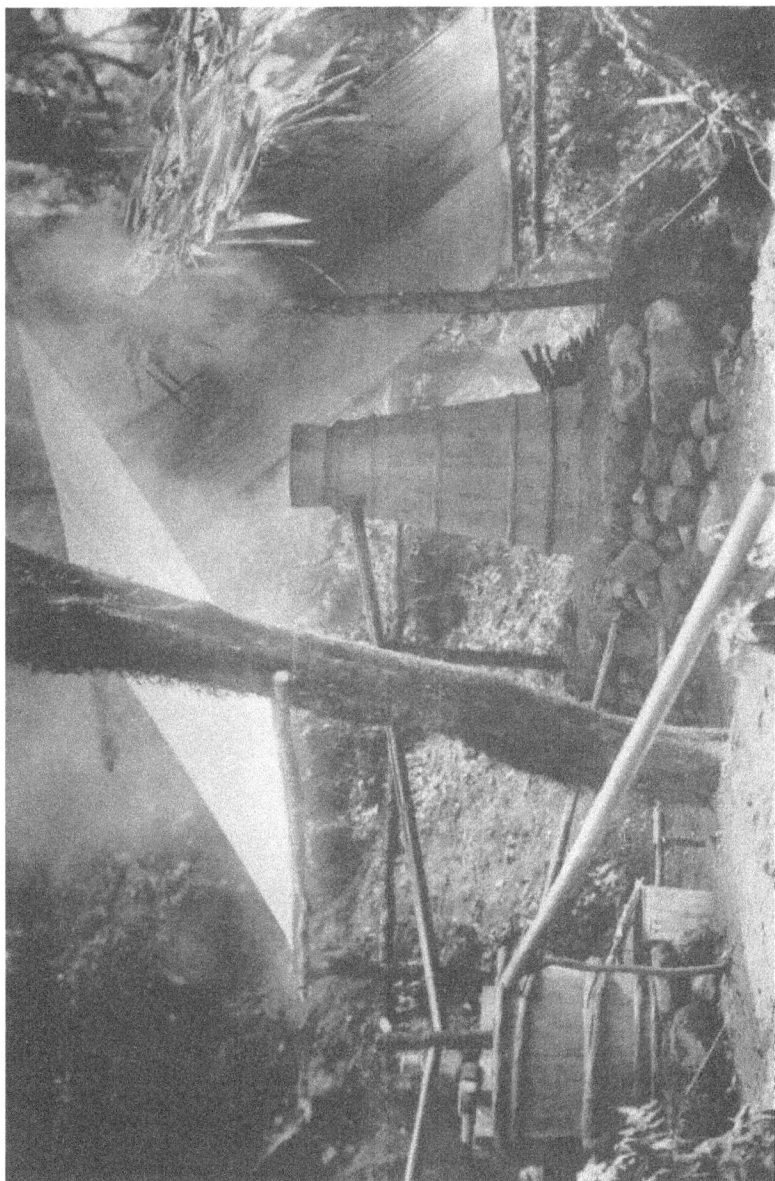

Distillation of *Shô-Gjū* oil at *Heishana.*

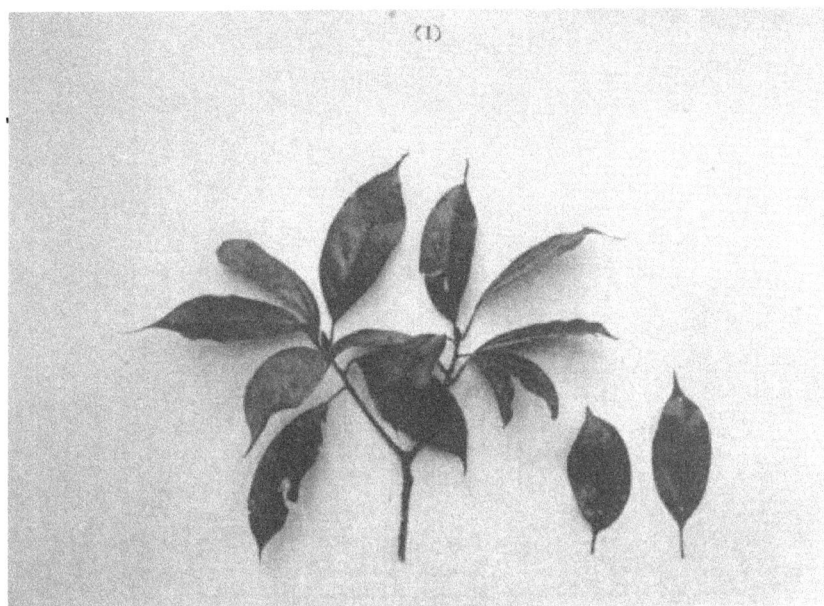

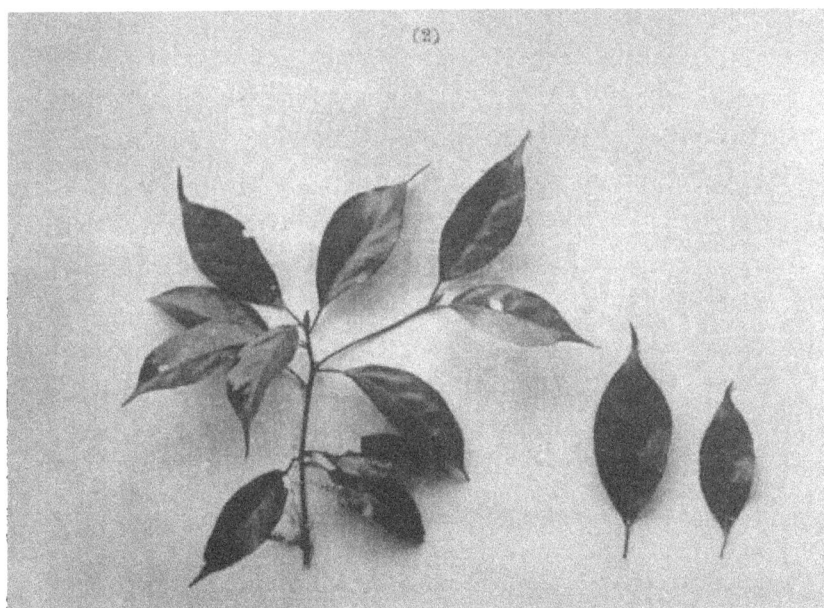

Leaves of *Shô-Gyŭ.*—(1) From *Arisan,* (2) from *Tebutegai.*

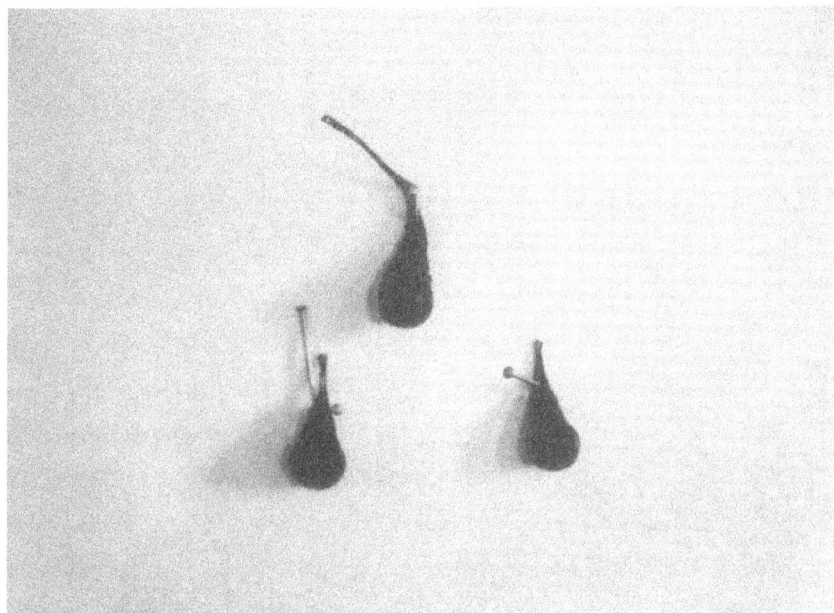

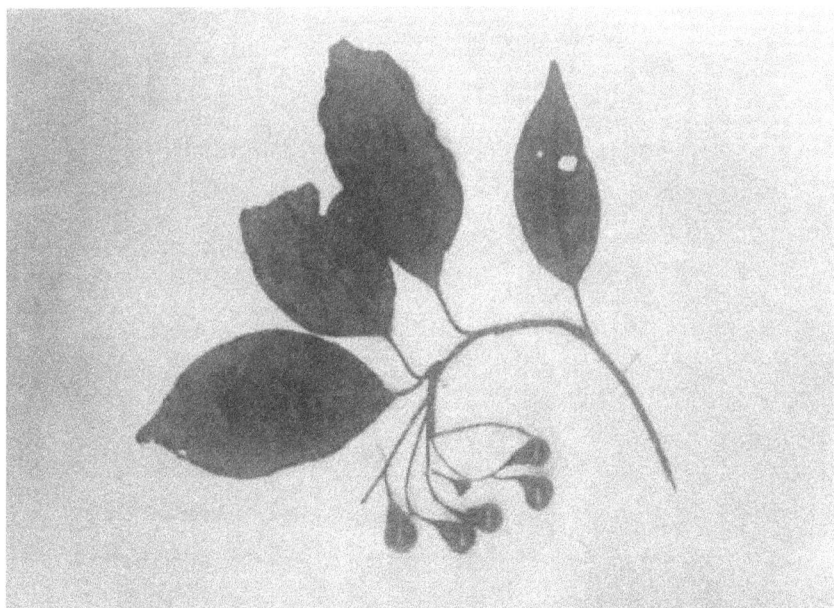

Leaves and fruit of *Shô-Gyū* tree in *Shinchiku.*

CONTENTS.

	PAGE
Shô-Gyū Oil and the Shô-Gyū Tree ··· ··· ··· ··· ··· ··· ··· ···	1
Growing Districts of Shô-Gyū Trees and their Location ··· ··· ···	3
Method Employed in the Preparation of Shô-Gyū Oil ··· ··· ···	6
Yield of Shô-Gyū Oil ··· ··· ··· ··· ··· ··· ··· ··· ··· ··· ···	7
Total Production of Shô-Gyū Oil ··· ··· ··· ··· ··· ··· ··· ···	9
Physical Properties of Shô-Gyū Oil ··· ··· ··· ··· ··· ··· ··· ···	10
Examination of Shô-Gyū Oil by Distillation ··· ··· ··· ··· ··· ···	12
Acid and Ester Values of Shô-Gyū Oil ··· ··· ··· ··· ··· ··· ···	16
Determination of Total Alcohol Contained in Shô-Gyū Oil ··· ···	18
Constituents of Shô-Gyū Oil ··· ··· ··· ··· ··· ··· ··· ··· ···	20
1. Formaldehyde ··· ··· ··· ··· ··· ··· ··· ··· ··· ··· ···	20
2. Sabinene ··· ··· ··· ··· ··· ··· ··· ··· ··· ··· ··· ···	21
3. Dipentene ··· ··· ··· ··· ··· ··· ··· ··· ··· ··· ···	24
4. a - terpinene ··· ··· ··· ··· ··· ··· ··· ··· ··· ···	25
5. γ - terpinene ··· ··· ··· ··· ··· ··· ··· ··· ··· ···	25
Linalool ··· ··· ··· ··· ··· ··· ··· ··· ··· ··· ···	25
6. Terpinenol - 4 ··· ··· ··· ··· ··· ··· ··· ··· ··· ···	26
7. Geraniol ··· ··· ··· ··· ··· ··· ··· ··· ··· ··· ···	33
8. Citronellol ··· ··· ··· ··· ··· ··· ··· ··· ··· ··· ···	34
9. Safrol ··· ··· ··· ··· ··· ··· ··· ··· ··· ··· ···	34
10. Eugenol ··· ··· ··· ··· ··· ··· ··· ··· ··· ··· ···	35
Cadinene ··· ··· ··· ··· ··· ··· ··· ··· ··· ··· ···	35
The Value of Shô-Gyū Oil as an Essential Oil ··· ··· ··· ··· ···	36

Abbreviations.

d = specific gravity.

$d_{15°}$ = specific gravity at 15° C.

$a_{D15°}$ = optical rotation at 15° C, in a 100 mm. tube.

$n_{D20°}$ = index of refraction at 20° C.

B. p. = boiling point.

b. p. $t°$ (7 mm.) = boiling point $t°$ C. at 7 mm. pressure.

M. p. = melting point.

g. = gram.

cc. = cubic centimetre.

mm. = millimetre.

Shô-Gyū Oil and the Shô-Gyū Tree.

"*Shô-Gyū* Oil" is the name given to an essential oil with an aromatic odour, distilled from a perennial tree popularly called by the natives "*Chiuⁿ-Gû*,"[*] growing chiefly in the highland forest regions of Formosa. On account of its not producing camphor through the regular process of manufacture, the *Chiuⁿ-Gû* (*Shô-Gyū*), the source of the oil, has played so far a very insignificant part in the industrial world, utterly failing to draw the attention of those connected with the industry. While the *Shô-Gyū* tree exhibits some features in common with the *Shiu-Shô* tree[†], as in the lack of solid camphor or in other superficial indications, the latter luxuriates in the camphor-tree regions and has aroused wide public interest as a highly valuable material for industrial researches; whereas the former, thriving exclusively in an isolated region beyond that of the camphor tree, was completely overlooked, and even the essential oil it produces has hardly been the subject of discussion.

Seen at a distance, the *Shô-Gyū* tree presents a strong resemblance to the camphor tree. The natives in the locality of *Kōsempo* (*Kah-sien-po*) call it "*Gû-Chiuⁿ*," a term presumably corrupted from the savage tongue. At the present stage of investigation, however, its scientific name and classification are still a matter of conjecture and doubt, but, following the opinion of Dr. Hayata based upon several specimens collected in *Kōsempo*, *Taiko* (*Tai-fu*), and *Arisan* (*Ali-soaⁿ*) districts, we may assume that it belongs to the Laurineæ. The "black camphor" tree, as it is generally called by the manufacturers of camphor, appears to be the same tree.

---

*. *Chiu^u* or *Shô* (樟) = camphor tree; *Gû* or *Gyû* (牛) = ox.

† *Shiu* (臭) = stinking.

There is, however, no proof of the assumption, nor has any report ever
been made regarding the collection of its flowers,—the blooming season is
said to be from February to March; hence it is evidently impossible to
determine its scientific name. In view of a future study of a collection
of flower specimens, the discussions are restricted here to the scope of
external forms. The following are the results of observations made on
the tree as it flourishes in the thick woods along the length of the old
Arisan road (*Kî-koan-tài*) in *Kagi* (*Ka-gî*) prefecture, and in the vicinity
of *Heishana* (*Piêng-chia-nâ*)— a mountainous region extending from a
locality popularly called "*Cross road*" (*Chap-jî-lö*) up to the elevated
region of *Arisan*, where conifers thrive.

The trunk of the *Shô-Gyū* tree usually attains a height of 40 to 50
shaku,* the circumference of the larger ones often measuring, at a man's
height, from 15 to 20 *shaku*; and the growth of the tree is, speaking
generally, uniform and vigorous with no dwarfed specimens. The greater
portion of the trunk is generally covered with-lichens and mosses, with a
few exceptions where the bark is much exposed; also, many are entwined
by vines and climbers. The bark, when compared with that of the
camphor tree, suggests at a glance a somewhat brownish-red colour.
The large branches have smooth longitudinal wrinkles and furrows upon
the greyish-white surface. A piece of *Shô-Gyū* wood from *Tebutegai* was
found equally covered with lichens and other parasites in spots upon
the bark, displaying identical features in its external peculiarities with
specimens from *Arisan*. The longitudinal section of the branch shows
that the heartwood seems rather white in comparison with that of the
camphor, *Shiu-Shô*, or *Yu-Ju* tree. The wood is soft and sappy, seemingly
containing much moisture, and the solidity naturally failing to equal that
of the camphor tree, it can be sawed or chopped with comparatively little
exertion. Despite the extreme difficulty of distinguishing the tree from

* 1 *shaku* = 0·994 ft. = 0·303 m.

the camphor tree by mere observation of external appearances in the living states, the test can readily be accomplished by shaving small pieces from the sapwood portion—particularly the root—of the two trees, and judging from their inherent odour. This test has incidentally proved to be the most reliable method of detecting the difference between the two. A simpler method, however, is the examination of the leaves. The leaves of the *Shô-Gyū* tree have a bright deep-green colour upon the surface and are much thicker than those of the camphor tree, (a large one often measuring about 13 cm. in length, and 4·5 cm. in width), and are slender in form with a particularly pointed apex which frequently reaches a length of 1 cm. On examination of a speciemen collected in November, a large terminal leaf-bud about 1 cm. in length and 0·5 cm. in diameter was found on the upper end of every young branch, by observation of which the tree may also be distinguished from the camphor tree. The latter test, however, being only practicable when the shoots with leaves attached are within reach, it is highly advisable to employ the former test at the same time, in order to insure a correct determination.

Growing Districts of *Shô-Gyū* Trees, and their Location.

Although the investigations regarding the geographical distribution of the *Shô-Gyū* tree have not yet covered the entire island, the regions where the tree grows are approximately ascertained from the practical survey carried out in three prefecture— *Shinchiku* (*Sin-tek*), *Kagi*, and *Akō* (*A-kâu*)— and the total existing stocks are estimated at an enormous amount. The following are concise descriptions of the prevailing conditions relative to the *Shô-Gyū*-growing districts in the prefectures just mentioned.

4)

In the prefecture of *Akō* there are remarkably rich districts in the division of *Kōsempo*, especially in the locality of *Tebutegai*. A tract of land, several miles in length, extending from Valley No. 1 to No. 6, is considered to be one of the best districts in that vicinity. According to the statements of Mr. T. Nagai, of the Sakurai Camphor Distillery in *Kōsempo*, the existing stocks of camphor and *Shō-Gyū* trees in the localities of *Tebutegai* are in an approximate proportion of three to seven. The late Mr. Shida, a delegated official of the Savages' Department of the Formosan Government, asserted that, on his descending trip from Mount *Shimbôrei* (*Sin-bōng-niâ*) in connection with the reconnoisance survey, the trees he observed along the entire distance, to cover which took from 7 A.M. to 3 P.M., were the *Shō-Gyū* only, thus indicating an exceptionally rich store of the timber. Continuing his previous statement, Mr. Nagai said that the investigations relating to the camphor-producing industry having been completed as far as Valley No. 6, *Tebutegai*, not only was the presence of *Shō-Gyū* in intermediate localities confirmed, but the extent of its growth in the elevated regions along the *Namasen-kei* (*Lâm-chú-sien R.*) up to Mount Morrison, could also be inferred from the conditions prevailing in other growing districts, together with the information furnished by the aborigines. In conclusion, he remarked that, owing to the supposed existence of the *Shō-Gyū* tree, which is very likely to be mistaken for the camphor tree, because of its close resemblance to the latter in external form, only one hundred and twenty furnaces instead of the original three hundred, were erected sometime ago in Valley No. 6, *Tebutegai*. These authentic statements may well be accepted as data to establish the existence of the tree in the regions mentioned above. In addition, Mr. Tadokoro, head of *Kōsempo* division of the prefecture, holds a similar opinion in regard to its existence in a luxuriant state in the mountain region beyond *Tebutegai* in the south of *Shimbôrei*, at an altitude of about 5,000 *shaku*, which forms the water-shed between *Rokkiri* (*Lak-ku-li*) and *Kōsempo* divisions of the prefecture.

In *Kagi* prefecture there are dense forests of *Shô-Gyū* covering vast regions. According to Mr. Ichikawa of the Utsunomiya Camphor Distillery, the existence of similar forests is equally confirmed in regions along the upper course of the *Suisan-kei* (*Chúi-soaⁿ-khoe*), in the vicinity of the fountain-head of *Sekisuisan-kei* (*Chiô-chúi soaⁿ-khoe*), as well as in the neighbouring districts of *Chokoban-kei* (*Chiô-phíⁿ-pôaⁿ-khoe*) that borders *Nantō* (*Lâm-tâu*) prefecture. The information he received is further assurance of their existence in many parts of the wild regions in *Nantō* prefecture.

The *Taiko* division of *Shinchiku* prefecture and the neighbouring locality have the distinction of being the original quarter where the oil employed as material in the present studies was produced; also of being the quarter where the discovery of the tree was first reported. Summing up the results of various investigations, the *Shô-Gyū*-growing districts in this prefecture seem to cover an immense area. According to the personal investigations carried out by Mr. R. Tashiro, an official expert of the Monopoly Bureau, a certain section of *Denshōsan* (*Chhân-sieng-soaⁿ*) in the neighbourhood of *Ritōsan* (*Lõe-thau-soaⁿ*) in *Jukirin* (*Su-ki-lim*) division of the prefecture, is so thickly covered with the trees that it seems at a distance to be a vast mass of the pure *Shô-Gyū* forest. Good prospects are further promised in the regions of *Yurasan* (*Iu-lo-san*) and *Karizensan* (*Ka-li-chiang-san*), not to speak of *Kita-Sensuisan* (*Pak-sôe-chúi-soaⁿ*) and *Nishi-Sensuisan* (*Sai-sôe-chúi-soaⁿ*), which embrace rich forests of the tree.

From these facts it is plainly seen that the *Shô-Gyū*-growing districts are numerous and extensive in the aforementioned three prefectures, which will be substantially multiplied, in case the so-called black camphor tree is proved to be the *Shô-Gyū*; and, finally, should the *Shô-Gyū* districts be found to form a chain or to be distributed over the whole island, their combined area would, indeed, comprise a prodigious tract. ·

Judging from the actual investigations of the growing districts, the *Shô-Gyū* tree appears to be a perennial thriving in highland regions in continuous groups, forming a distinctly independent belt, and entirely differing from the *Shiu-Shô* tree, which grows wildly in the camphor regions. Speaking of its geographical distribution with reference to the existing conditions in *Arisan*, no trace of the tree, except in wild forests, is seen for a distance of some hundred yards along the hill road of the *Arisan* camphor district; in the region beyond that, however, dense forests of the tree are located. In other words, the tree begins to make its appearance at an altitude of about 5,000 *shaku*, extending up to 6,500 *shaku*, and then disappears, giving way to the conifers. Hence the formation in concentrated groups seems to be one of the striking characteristics of the tree. In the surrounding localities of *Heishana*, *Arisan*, large trees are noted, in groups of three and five, standing almost perfectly straight, and displaying magnificent forms of the trunks, which give one a lasting impression of beauty and grandeur. There is a considerable number of the trees in these woods with the upper portion of the trunk broken off by storms, some having decayed with age and fallen.

Method Employed in the Preparation of *Shô-Gyū* Oil.

The method of producing *Shô-Gyū* oil is much simpler than that of preparing camphor oil, on account of the absence of stearoptene. The entire operating outfit and equipments required in mountain districts for the preparation of *Shiu* oil are directly utilizable. The principal part of the apparatus consists of the *Tosa* tank or still to which a condenser, in the form of a spiral pipe, is attached. The steam and the oil liberated on distillation are condensed in passing through it, and the latter is collected in a receiver constructed on the principle of the *Florentine* flask*.

Yield of *Shô-Gyū* Oil.

Considering the results of an experimental preparation of the oil in *Kita-sensuisan* division of *Shinchiku* prefecture, the yield was estimated at an average of about 2·5% of the wood used. The test with the only wood obtained at Valley No. 2, *Tebutegai*, through the courtesy of Mr. Tadokoro, showed a yield of about 3·0%. Further experiments with the oils distilled in *Arisan* and *Kôsempo* resulted in a yield of 1·3 to 3·0%. The following tables give a brief account of the above experiments, together with the circumference and length of the trunk used, etc.

1. *Shô-Gyū* oils distilled in *Kita-sensuisan.*

TABLE SHOWING THE RESULTS OF EXPERIMENTAL PREPARATION.

(The experiments were conducted by Mr. Tashiro, an expert, at the Camphor Distillery No. 17 in *Sensuisan.*)

No.	Variety	*Shô-Gyū* tree used as material		Specific gravity of wood at 20°			Results of distillation		Percentage of oil produced
		Circumference at a man's height	Length of trunk	Sapwood	Heartwood	Root	Quantity of chips used	Quantity of oil distilled	
		shaku	*shaku*				*mounme†*	*mounme*	
1	Living tree	13·8	43	1·024	1·007	1·007	211,390	5,667	2·68
2	"	15·8	42	1·034	1·049	1·043	45,700	812	1·78
3	"	14·0	60	0·882	0·968	1·041	46,570	1,016	2·18

* Detailed descriptions of the distilling apparatus are given in " Studies of *Shiu* Oil."

† 1 *mounme* = { 2·12 drams (Avoir.) / 2·41 dwts. (Troy.) } = 3·75 grms.

(Continued.)

4	Living tree	15·6	36	0·949	1·027	1·041	51,200	1,018	1·98
5	"	11·3	54	0·920	1·071	1·079	54,740	1,137	2·08
6	Fallen tree	9·3	42	—	—	—	36,170	1,180	3·26
7	Living tree	7·5	24	1·006	0·993	1·045	44,980	1,130	2·45
8	"	10·7	36	0·914	1·071	1·079	224,040	6,684	2·98
9	"	15·0	69	1·024	1·145	1·136	39,000	738	1·89
10	"	10·5	54	0·940	0·909	1·103	39,200	513	1·31

2. *Shô-Gyū* oil obtained from a tree grown in *Tebutegai.*

TABLE SHOWING THE RESULT OF EXPERIMENTAL PREPARATION.

(Conducted by the Department of Production of the Monopoly Bureau in *Taihoku.*)

			momme	*grm.*	
Living tree	Produced by distilling with steam for 23 hours, 55 minutes.		1,785	206	3·08

3. *Shô-Gyū* oils distilled in *Arisan.*

TABLE SHOWING THE RESULTS OF EXPERIMENTAL PREPARATION.

No.	Shô-Gyū tree used as material		Results of distillation		Percentage of oil produced
	Diameter at a man's height	Length of trunk from the ground to the lowest branch	Quantity of chips used	Quantity of oil distilled	
	shaku	*ken**	*kwan†*	*momme*	
1	3·2	8·0	354·400	5,920	1·57
2	3·0	5·0	38·500	530	1·38
3	4·3	4·5	47·000	595	1·27
4	2·8	5·0	44·800	1,320	2·95
5	4·0	6·0	360·720	5,335	1·48
6	2·6	7·0	247·000	5,205	2·11

* 1 *ken* = 6 *shaku* = 1·99 yds. = 1·82 metres.

† 1 *kwan* = 1000 *momme* = $\left\{ \begin{array}{l} 8\cdot27 \text{ lbs. (Avoir.)} \\ 10\cdot05 \text{ lbs. (Troy.)} \end{array} \right\}$ = 3·75 kilograms.

4. *Shô-Gyū* oils prepared at Valley No. 2, *Tebutegai.*

TABLE SHOWING THE RESULTS OF EXPERIMENTAL PREPARATION.

No.	Circumference at a man's height	Length of trunk from the ground to the lowest branch	Quantity of chips used	Quantity of oil distilled	Percentage of oil produced
	shaku	*ken*	*kwan*	*momme*	
1	11·0	8·0	41·400	1,040	2·51
3	18·5	4·5	269·000	6,485	2·41
4	18·0	9·0	257·620	5,266	2·04
5	23·5	7·0	53·100	760	1·43
8	9·0	6·0	48·500	1,004	2·07
13	9·5	10·0	277·800	4,696	1·69

Total Production of *Shô-Gyū* Oil.

Despite the difficulty at the present empirical stage of determining the exact figures of the total output of *Shô-Gyū* oil, an approximate estimate may be made, following the opinions of the manufacturers of camphor, who have investigated the rich resources of this product. " It is unanimously conceded by experts," remarked Mr. Nagai, " that the vast tract stretching within a radius of 3 *ri** with Valley No. 1 in *Tebutegai* as its centre, is exceedingly rich in *Shô-Gyū* trees, and I am inclined to say that an annual production of 600,000 *kin* would not be improbable." Mr. Ichikawa, manager of the Camphor Department of Messrs. Utsunomiya & Co. in *Kagi* prefecture, has also intimated that, with the installation of one hundred furnaces in that prefecture, an output of 240,000 to 300,000 *kin* per annum as a conservative estimate is promised, figuring on a minimum yield of 2%. It is also, unquestionably, the accepted opinion that a large production in the prefecture of

* 1 *ri* = 2·44 miles = 3·93 kilometres.

Shinchiku is promised when disturbances cease and peace reigns in the savage districts.

Physical Properties of Shô-Gyu Oil.

Shô-Gyū oil contains a remarkably large number of chemical components, its known constituents being not less than ten ; and as their proportion differs according to the properties that the individual tree possesses, so the physical properties of the oil are naturally affected. When two varieties of the oil possessing properties farthest apart are compared, they frequently appear to differ apparently in chemical nature, but their identification is established by the odour peculiar to this oil.

Colour.—The oil is usually colourless, or has a light yellow or yellow colour,* and on account of its stability against decomposition, it may be stored for a long period with little fear of coloration or chemical change.

Specific gravity.—Judging from the numerous specimens collected, the specific gravity of the oil appears to vary somewhat widely according to their place of origin. The lightest variety of the *Shinchiku* product had as low a gravity as 0·900, while the heaviest of the *Arisan* showed 1·031.

Optical rotation.—The oil has a dextrorotary power throughout all the varieties, the minimum figure being $a_{D9°}+7·75°$. An experiment with the only specimen from *Kōsempo* showed an intensity of over $+30°$.

Refractive index.—This constant also fluctuates concomitantly with the other constants, the minimum value being about 1·4750. The following are the results obtained from the examination of these specimens :—

---

* Oil No. 6 produced in *Arisan* had a bright red colour — a very rare instance.

Place of origin	No.	Colour	d at t°		a_D at t°		n_D at t°		Odour	Colour-reaction with mercuric sulphate
Shinchiku	1	Faint yellow	0·908	9	+ 29·50	5	1·47753	20½	Slightly resembling oil of savin	Trace ?
"	2	Colourless	0·910	"	+ 23·25	"	1·47478	19½	Sweetish, and as that of No. 1	+
"	3	Light yellow	0·911	"	+ 15·88	"	1·47468	20	Same as No. 1	Trace ?
"	4	"	0·931	"	+ 14·90	"	1·48713	18	"	+
"	5	Colourless	0·912	"	+ 24·55	"	1·47567	20	Recalling oil of nutmeg	+
"	6	Faint yellow	0·900	"	+ 23·50	"	1·47665	19	—	+
"	7	"	0·927	"	+ 22·30	"	1·48133	20	—	+
"	8	Colourless	0·945	"	+ 18·50	"	1·48471	20½	—	+
"	9	Faint yellow	0·933	"	+ 15·25	"	1·48094	20	—	Trace ?
"	10	"	0·914	"	+ 22·20	"	1·47694	19	—	+·
Kosempo	—	Yellow	0·910	11	+ 34·45	11	1·48326	"	Reminding of oil of nutmeg	+
Arisan	1	Light yellow	0·968	25	+ 12·83	25	1·49466	26	—	Trace ?
"	2	Faint yellow	0·939	"	+ 14·40	"	1·48490	25½	—	(?)
"	3	Light yellow	0·993	26	+ 8·55	26	1·50088	25	—	Trace ?
"	4	Almost colourless	0·949	"	+ 16·65	25	1·48971	"	—	"
"	5	"	0·993	"	+ 13·25	"	1·50227	"	—	+
"	6	Bright red	0·925	25	+ 12·40	"	1·47912	"	Recalling oil of sweet marjoram	.(?)
Tebutegai	1	Faint yellow	0·943	"	+ 19·31	25½	1·48971	"	—	+
"	3	Light yellow	0·970	26	+ 16·25	"	1·49693	25½	—	(?)
"	4	Faint yellow	1·030	"	+ 7·75	26	1·51302	25	—	+
"	5	Light yellow	0·993	"	+ 11·05	"	1·50237	"	Reminding of oil of nutmeg	Trace ?
"	8	"	0·965	"	+ 13·34	"	1·49429	"	—	+
"	13	"	0·908	"	+ 24·25	"	1·47987	"	—	+

Examination of *Shô-Gyū* Oil by Distillation.

I. SHINCHIKU OILS.

No. 1. No. 2.

Boiling point	Percentage proportion	d at t°		α_D at t°		Percentage proportion	d at t°		α_D at t°	
Up to 185°	32.88	0.874	10	+38.75	10½	10.08	0.873	13	+26.50	13
185 — 195°	24.64	0.884	10½	+31.00	11	32.80	0.889	"	+24.15	15
195 — 205°	13.60	0.9215	11	+23.30	"	26.40	0.914	14	+22.25	14
205 — 215°	23.68	0.950	12	+20.30	12	25.84	0.9375	"	+24.25	"
Residue	5.20	—		—		4.88	—		—	

No. 3. No. 5.

Boiling point	Percentage proportion	d at t°		α_D at t°		Percentage proportion	d at t°		α_D at t°	
Up to 185°	16.08	0.888	13	+14.12	13	17.52	0.875	11	+33.28	12
185 — 195°	39.20	0.8925	"	+14.25	"	26.56	0.886	12	+27.75	"
195 — 205°	17.56	0.915	14	+17.20	"	22.32	0.914	"	+21.00	"
205 — 215°	21.76	0.940	"	+20.20	15	28.80	0.946	"	+21.92	"
Residue	5.40	—		—		4.80	—		—	

No. 7. No. 9.

Boiling point	Percentage proportion	d at t°		α_D at t°		Percentage proportion	d at t°		α_D at t°	
Up to 185°	8.48	0.878	10	+32.12	10	4.16	0.895	11½	+15.44	11½
185 — 195°	31.52	0.890	"	+28.00	"	26.00				
195 — 205°	16.32	0.909	11	+21.88	"	28.24	0.915	"	+15.87	"
205 — 215°	29.36	0.954	"	+19.75	11	24.24	0.953	12	+17.50	12
Residue	14.32	1.007	"	+12.07	"	17.36	1.005	"	+11.58	"

No. 4.　　　No. 8.

Up to 185°	1·12	0·895	12	+18·70	12	2·72	0·894	12	+23·68	12
185 — 195°	19·60					19·36				
195 — 205°	22·64	0·912	//	+16·70	12½	25·12	0·917	//	+20·65	//
205 — 215°	26·08	0·955	12½	+15·75	//	30·40	0·955	11½	+18·50	11½
215 — 225°	24·88	1·007	13	+11·81	13	18·40	1·006	//	+14·35	//
Residue	5·68	—		—		4·00	—		—	

No. 6.　　　No. 10.

Up to 185°	5·40	—		+26·35	10	10·40	0·876	12	+27·25	12
185 — 195°	33·00	0·889	10	+24·45	//	35·20	0·890	//	+24·14	//
195 — 205°	29·40	0·911	//	+23·00	//	22·48	0·914	//	+20·40	//
205 — 215°	29·04	0·938	//	+25·08	//	27·12	0·946	//	+20·92	//
Residue	3·16	—		—		4·80	—		—	

II. KŌSEMPO OIL.

Up to 175°	18·00	0·862	10	+52·85	10
175 — 185°	33·60	0·868	//	+47·50	//
185 — 195°	10·40	0·886	//	+35·85	9½
195 — 205°	6·88	0·908	//	+24·09	//
205 — 215°	6·58	—		+13·55	//
Residue	24·56	1·039	//	+ 4·16	//

III. Arisan Oils.

No. 3.   No. 4.

	No. 3					No. 4				
Up to 185°	5·60	—		+15·12	26	6·96	—		+29·00	25
185 — 195°						18·00	0·889	25	+25·75	"
195 — 205°	18·00	0·917	26	+13·12	"	23·20	0·905	"	+20·40	"
205 — 215°	17·44	0·950	"	+11·25	"	10·00	0·954	"	+14·25	"
215 — 225°	28·48	1·012	"	+8·50	"	33·60	1·005	"	+10·65	"
225 — 235°	27·68	1·065	"	+2·80	"	8·24	1·064	"	+1·25	"
Residue	2·80	—		—						

No. 6.

Up to 185°	18·80	0·880	26	+15·15	26
185 — 195°	24·80	0·890	"	+13·75	"
195 — 205°	15·60	0·909	"	+12·50	"
205 — 215°	16·56	0·952	"	+12·57	"
215 — 220°	10·80	0·981	"	+11·40	"
Residue	13·44	1·030	"	—	

IV. Tebutegai Oils.

No. 1.   No. 13.

	No. 1					No. 13				
Up to 185°	10·40	0·870	26	+36·00	26	31·20	0·863	26½	+36·40	26½
185 — 195°	19·76	0·885	"	+30·62	"	20·80	0·875	26	+29·75	26
195 — 205°	17·76	0·906	26½	+23·25	26½	14·50	0·900	"	+18·32	"
205 — 215°	15·44	0·948	27	+15·30	27	16·40	0·950	"	+13·00	"
215 — 220°	23·76	1·010	"	+9·25	"	17·10	1·014	27	+8·16	27
Residue	12·88	1·058	"	+2·00	"					

No. 3.   No. 4.

	No. 3					No. 4				
Up to 185°	4·00	0·885	27	+30·62	27	10·40	0·920	26½	+22·64	26½
185 — 195°	20·00									
195 — 205°	9·20	0·904	"	+23·70	"					
205 — 215°	12·24	0·950	"	+16·30	"	14·00	0·963	"	+14·20	"
215 — 225°	36·48	1·010	"	+10·55	"	25·84	1·017	"	+ 8·00	"
225 — 231°	18·08	1·070	"	+ 2·60	"	44·40	1·075	"	+ 2·20	"
Residue						5·36	—		—	

Considering the state of fractionation resulting from the above experiments, it will be seen that the terpene fractions or those below 205° are generally moderate in quantity, while those above 215° are comparatively small, except in the case of heavy oils. The specific gravity of terpene fractions gradually falls through a single process of fractional distillation, and at the same time the optical rotation is noted to rise readily. Some fractions up to 185° showed a remarkable rise of over +10°; especially the first fraction of the *Kōsempo* product exhibited the highest rotation of +52°, whereas the fractions boiling between 195—205° of the *Shinchiku* products Nos. 2, 5, 6 and 10 were seen to fall in rotation. Regarding the oils of this nature, a test was made for the colour reaction of linalool, to which references were given in "Studies of *Shiu* Oil."* In the case of *Shiu* oil,

---

* According to several magazines and publications on essential oils, *Shiu* oil is frequently treated under the assumed name of "*Apopin* oil", but this term presumably owes its origin to "*Amoping*" (阿姆坪), where the oil was once experimentally prepared. Mr. Keimatsu attributes its source to "*Anping*" (安平), which is, however, highly doubtful. Since the oil has been familiarly known as "*Shiu* oil", attempts to disseminate and popularize it under the name of "*Apopin* oil" would ultimately result in failure. As regards "*Apopinol*", the so-called new terpene alcohol of *Apopin* oil, it may be interesting to mention here that the alcohol stands almost on the same footing in the principle of nomenclature as "*Camphorogenol*" in camphor oil, and apopinol, being nothing but a mixture of d-camphor and l-linalool, never occurs in *Shiu* oil except in *Apopin* oil. Further details concerning this alcohol are given in "Studies of *Shiu* oil" compiled by the Bureau in 1912.

the test gives a satisfactory result. But *Shô-Gyū* oil, on being simply shaken with Denigès's reagent, produces no distinct coloration, which is perhaps due to the extremely small proportion of linalool contained. As the most reliable method, therefore, 7—10 cc. of the reagent is warmed to a temperature of about 50°, and 0.3—0.5 cc. of the test oil is subsequently added; then the whole liquid is slightly shaken three or four times, and the change of colour between two layers is immediately observed. If a small proportion of linalool be present, a red ring is formed between the layers; in case, however, the characteristic red colour fails to appear, it should be borne in mind that the coloration is often accelerated by slightly warming the upper layer over a Bunsen burner flame. Even a small quantity of linalool contained in several essential oils being detected by this reaction, all the *Shô-Gyū* oils in hand were tested in a similar manner. The results of examination showed that the coloration of the fractions. (b. p. 195—205°) with low optical activity was exceptionally plain and distinct. *Shinchiku* oils Nos. 1, 3, 7 and 9, however, produced only a slight reaction.

Since the foregoing process is merely an application of the test for the linalool colour-reaction on *Shô-Gyū* oil, a further examination is necessary in order to determine whether some other substances likely to produce a similar reaction are present. Even admitting the presence of linalool, its proportion being, it seems, exceedingly small, the examination will be resumed on the acquisition of sufficient material.

Acid and Ester Values of *Shô-Gyū* Oil.

Shô-Gyū oil as well as *Shiu* oil generally has only a slight acidity and a small ester value, the latter of which may be considered as a notable feature of some Formosan essential oils produced from the Laurineæ.

Origin	No.	Acid value	Ester value	Saponification value
Taiko	1	0·15	0·75	0·90
"	2	(1) 0·63 (2) 0·63	(1) 0·65 —	(1) 1·28 —
"	3	0·43	0·21	0·64
"	4	0·46	0·78	1·24
"	5	0·26	0·99	1·25
"	6	0·42	0·57	0·99
"	7	0·41	0·91	1·32
"	8	0·96	1·18	1·87
"	9	(1) 0·87 (2) 0·82	— (2) 0·43	— (2) 1·25
"	10	0·62	0·84	1·46
Kōsempo	—	0·10	0·59	0·69
Arisan	3	0·30	0·00	0·30
"	4	(1) 0·59 (2) 0·55	(1) 2·40 (2) 2·25	(1) 2·99 (2) 2·80
"	6	0.71	0·42	1·13
Tebutegai	1	(1) 0·44 (2) 0·47	(1) 0·41 —	(1) 0·85 —
"	4	(1) 0·21 (2) 0·20	(1) 0·00 —	(1) 0·21 —
"	13	0·76	1·09	1·85

Solubility of *Shô-Gyū* Oil in Alcohol.

Origin	No.	Solubility in alcohol of	
		80%	90%
		Room-temp. = 30°	
Shinchiku	1	1 : 1·20 vol.	1 : 0·35 vol.
"	2	1 : 1·00 "	1 : 0·22 "
"	3	1 : 0·98 "	—
"	4	1 : 1·00 "	1 : 0·31 "
"	5	1 : 0·95 "	1 : 0·23 "
"	6	1 : 1·00 "	—
"	7	1 : 1·05 "	1 : 0·32 "

Shinchiku	8	1 :	0·98 vol.	—
"	9	1 :	0·98 "	1 : 0·29 vol.
"	10	1 :	1·00 "	—
Kōsempo	—	1 :	12·50* "	1 : 0·51 "
Arisan	1	1 :	1·1 "	1 : 0·35 "
"	3	1 :	1·6 "	1 : 0·32 "
"	4	1 :	1·1 "	1 : 0·35 "
"	5	1 :	2·75 "	1 : 0·36 "
"	6	1 :	1·0 "	1 : 0·28 "
Tebutegai	1	1 :	1·45 "	1 : 0·35 "
"	3	1 :	1·6 "	1 : 0·35 "
"	4	1 :	4·35† "	1 : 0·38 "
"	5	1 :	2·85 "	1 : 0·35 "
"	13	1 :	1·3 "	1 : 0·37 "

Determination of Total Alcohol Contained in Shô-Gyū Oil.

For the quantitative determination of the alcohol-content of essential oils, the acetylation method, which customarily employs acetic anhydride and sodium acetate, is always adopted; but owing to partial decomposition of terpene alcohols, as well as the simultaneous formation of esterifiable substances from terpenes, which occurs during the process, it fails frequently, as is well known, to give accurate results, especially when applied to a test for oils containing various easily decomposable terpene alcohols, such as terpineol, linalool, and tertiary alcohols in general. Hence it must be understood that in the present experiments only approximate figures were obtainable, according to the properties of the oils under examination.

---

* Insoluble in 4 vol. of 80% alcohol with separation of 0·5 vol. of heavy oil-portion which clearly dissolves when highly diluted.

† Insoluble in 2·5 vol. of 80% alcohol with separation of heavy oil (0·5 vol.).

Origin	No.	d at t°		α_D at t°		Ester value after acetylation	Optical rotation of acetylated oil α_D at t°		Quantity of the original oil used	Quantity of sodium acetate	Quantity of acetic anhydride	Temp. of the oil-bath	Duration of acetylation	Time of saponification of acetylated oil
Taiko	1	0·908	9	+29·50°	9	84·1	—		10cc.	2 g.	10cc.	145 to 150°	2h	2h
"	2	0·910	"	+23·25°	"	100·7	—		"	"	"	"	"	"
"	5	0·912	"	+24·55°	"	(1) 77·5	—		"	"	"	146 to 147°	"	1·5
"	"	"	"	"	"	(2)105·6	—		"	"	"	"	"	2
"	8	0·945	"	+18·50°	"	(1) 75·5	—		"	"	"	"	"	1·5
"	"	"	"	"	"	(2) 81·9	—		"	"	"	"	"	2
Kōsempo	—	0·912	11	+34·45°	11	84·0	—		"	"	"	"	"	"
Taiko	3	0·911	9	+15·88°	9	101·6	+11·42°	14½	15cc.	"	20cc.	143 to 145°	"	"
"	6	0·900	"	+23·50°	"	(1) 85·7	+15·10°	15	"	"	"	"	"	1
"	"	"	"	"	"	(2) 94·8	—		"	"	"	"	"	2
"	9	0·933	"	+15·25°	"	(1) 58·2	+11·25°	15	"	"	"	"	"	1
"	"	"	"	"	"	(2) 71·5	—		"	"	"	"	"	2
"	4	0·951	"	+14·90°	"	105·0	+9·92°	10½	"	"	"	"	3	"
"	7	0·927	"	+22·30°	"	106·7	+11·25°	"	"	"	"	"	"	"
"	10	0·914	"	+22·20°	"	129·4	+11·43°	"	"	"	"	"	"	"
Arisan	3	0·993	26	+8·55°	26	(1) 52·2	—		"	"	"	"	"	1
"	"	"	"	"	"	(2) 62·2	—		"	"	"	"	"	2
"	4	0·949	"	+16·65°	25	81·7	—		"	"	"	"	"	"
"	6	0·929	25	+12·40°	"	94·5	—		"	"	"	"	"	"
Tebutegai	1	0·943	"	+19·31°	25½	83·1	—		"	"	"	142 to 143°	"	"
"	4	1·030	26	+7·75°	26	46·6	—		"	"	"	"	"	"
"	13	0·908	"	+24·25°	"	95·9	—		"	"	"	"	"	"

Calculated as $C_{10} H_{18} O$, the oil yields, provided the experiment be conducted properly, about 30 per cent. of alcohol, but the figures naturally vary according to the duration of acetylation and the time of saponification of the acetylated oil. Considering the fact that a prolonged saponification produces a comparatively good result, the presence of alcohol of terpineol type in this oil is presumable.

Constituents of Shô-Gyū Oil.

As has been shown in the first examination of the *Shinchiku* product on fractional distillation, the alcohol fractions that distil over after terpene fractions are fairly large in quantity, while those over 220° are comparatively small. Consequently, terpene and alcohol fractions are seen to represent the chief constituents of the oil, with the exception of heavy oils.

In other words, sabinene and terpinenol - 4 appear to form the main portion of the fraction. Besides these, there are also about eight different by-constituents, which were detected in the *Shinchiku* oils. Even the chief constituents are occasionally subject to variation according to the properties of original oils, certain varieties of which contain the by-constituents in excess of the principal. Oil No. 1, produced in *Shinchiku*, has been selected as the standard specimen for examination of the chemical properties of the oil, and the results of various tests with it are chiefly described in the following pages. Those of other specimens are also conveniently treated in the supplement.

(1) **Formaldehyde.**

The supposed presence of aldehyde of low fatty series, especially formaldehyde or acetaldehyde is a subject of conjecture and uncertainty, which is often met with during the course of examination of essential oils. In similar manner, the presence of certain substances which produce the characteristic aldehyde reaction in the first distillate of *Shô-Gyū* oil is noticeable. Their proportion, however, being exceedingly small, only the results of experiment for the colour-reaction, from which their presence may be assumed, are given below.

Properties of the liquid under examination	Vitali's reaction	Rimini's reaction	Decolourized fuchsine solution	Ammoniacal silver solution	Nessler's reagent	1% phloro-glucin sol. with NaOH
Distillation water obtained from oil No. 1 under diminished pressure	Bright brownish-red	Intense blue	Pale red	Deposited brownish precipitate	Immediately deposited brownish precipitate	Faintly purplish
The same obtained from oil No. 8	Brownish-red	Light brownish-yellow	—	—	—	—
Water deposited in the vessel containing oil No. 1	Pink-rose	Assumed a greenish-blue colour (but immediately disappeared)	Red	—	—	Claret-red

It may be understood from the above that oil No. 1 in the crude state produced Rimini's reaction, indicating the presence of form-aldehyde. Besides this, the oil produced in *Kösempo* gave in its first fraction a darkish-gray coloration with Denigès's reagent. As the available quantity of the oil was extremely small, it was impossible to proceed further with the test.

(2) Sabinene.

Oil No. 1 was first of all fractionated at reduced pressure (18 mm.), and split up into five approximately equal parts :—

Fraction	I.	$d_{22°}$ 0·858	$a_{D22°}$ + 33·90°*
"	II.	" 0·870	" + 27·80°
"	III.	" 0·893	" + 22·25°
"	IV.	" 0·936	" + 21·05°
"	V.	" 0·966	" + 17·00°

After a series of fractional distillation *in vacuo*, fraction I was again subjected to distillation at ordinary pressure, and the portion (b. p. 163—167°) was subdivided into the following fractions :—

B. p. 163—165°, $d_{12°}$ 0·8505, $a_{D12°}$ + 55·00°.

" 165—167°, $d_{11°}$ 0·8525, $a_{D11°}$ + 55·50°.

These fractions showed a tendency to increase in optical activity, but were turned into test-liquid on account of their limited quantity.

(A) Formation of sabinenic acid.

Oxidation with permanganate (24 g. of the fraction, 56 g. of potassium permanganate, 360 g. of water, 360 g. of ice, and 12 g. of caustic soda), according to Wallach's method, yielded principally sodium sabinenate which is sparingly soluble in water.

After filtration, it was recrystallised from water and the acid contained therein liberated. Recrystallised from dilute methyl alcohol, it showed the m. p. 57°, which agrees with that of sabinenic acid. The presence of sabinene in the original fraction was still further confirmed by the preparation of sabina-ketone from this acid.

---

* Refer to the table of fractional distillation.

(B) Formation of sabina-ketone.

The experiment was conducted with 30 g. of sodium sabinenate mentioned above, according to Wallach's method. The aqueous solution of sodium sabinenate, to which 10 cc. of dilute sulphuric acid had been added, was placed in a Martius flask provided with a separating funnel and proper fittings for steam distillation. The funnel was filled with a diluted permanganate solution previously acidulated with dilute sulphuric acid ; and, allowing the liquid to drop very slowly into the flask, a current of steam was transmitted at the same time, until the oxidation with permanganate was accomplished. The aqueous solution thus distilled over was saturated with common salt, followed by shaking together with ether, and after distilling off the latter from the solution, the remaining oil-portion was fractionally distilled at ordinary pressure. The resulting oil had an almost constant boiling point and was found to be exactly identical with sabina-ketone, its chief characteristics being :

B. p. 214—215° (uncorr.), $d_{19°} 0·956$, $\alpha_{D19°}-24·75°$, $n_{D22°} 1·46997$.

For the purpose of obtaining semicarbazone, it was further treated with semicarbazide hydrochloride in the usual manner, and the reaction mixture, after being repeatedly crystallized from methyl alcohol, yielded, as the product, sabina-ketone semicarbazone of the m. p. 140—141°.

A terpene fraction of the Kōsempo oil, possessing the properties : b. p. up to 175°, $d_{10°} 0·862$, $\alpha_{D10°}+52·85°$, when repeatedly fractionated, yielded an oil with the constants :

b. p. 162—164° $d_{17°} 0·8425$, $\alpha_{D17°}+64·00°$, $n_{D19°} 1·46731$,

which showed close agreement with pure sabinene in its properties.

a - pinene. In order to determine the presence of a-pinene in *Shô-Gyū* oil, a fraction (b. p. 158·5—160°, $d_{25°}$ 0·840, $a_{D25°}$ +47·40°), obtained from the first distillate, was tested for the preparation of pinene nitrosochloride, according to Wallach's method; but the result was negative. In cases, however, where a pinene fraction shows such a high rotation, it is generally recognized that the formation of nitrosochloride amounts to only a very small quantity, in spite of the presence of a-pinene. Hence, its presence can not be altogether denied because of this single manipulation. Further tests will be carried on later following Ehestädt's method or that of Agnew and Croad employing mercuric acetate.

Camphene. One of the first distillates having the properties: b. p. 160—162°, $d_{20°}$ 0·836, $a_{D20°}$ +48·10°, when tested for the presence of camphene by hydration according to Bertram and Walbaum's method, produced only a small quantity of an oily liquid with the odour of isoborneol.

(3) Dipentene.

When fraction II was repeatedly fractionated, the distillate boiling between 175—185° appeared to split up gradually into sabinene fraction and that of a higher boiling point than its own. Hence the smallest fraction boiling between 174—178° was examined for the preparation of dipentene-tetrabromide. Although small in bulk, it yet absorbed a moderate quantity of bromine. After standing for a few days, the syrupy reaction-product yielded the crystallised tetrabromide melting at 123—124°. Furthermore, by treating the original fraction with nitrosyl chloride, a nitrosochloride could be obtained, but this only appeared in extremely small quantities.

(4) and (5)   α - and ɤ - Terpinene.

The presence of terpinene in our *Shô-Gyū* oil, just as it occurs in Ceylon cardamom or marjoram oil in common with sabinene, was detected; but the simplest nitrosite test to determine the presence of α-terpinene appeared to be unsuccessful with *Shô-Gyū* oil. For the purpose of closer investigations, fraction III was subjected to a series of fractional distillation and the distillate boiling between 175—182°, when oxidised with alkaline permanganate under ice-cooling, afforded, as the resulting products, the erythritol, m. p. 236°, which proves the presence of ɤ-terpinene, and a small quantity of *i*-α·α′-dihydroxy-α-methyl-α′-isopropyl adipic acid, m. p. 188—189°, known as the derivative of α-terpinene. The latter was more closely identified from the corresponding dilactone, m. p. 73°. From these experiments the presence of terpinene, including α-as well as ɤ-terpinene, although in small quantity, was confirmed.

Linalool. As has been stated, the presence of linalool is presumable from the colour reaction with mercuric sulphate. But the distillate with a b. p. of 195—205°, obtained from a fraction of the *Shinchiku* oil No. 1, having failed to produce the colour reaction, it was repeatedly fractionated, which ultimately yielded the desired result. The proportion of linalool contained in the sample, however, appeared to be very small. Judging from the limits of the colour-reaction produced, the fractions with b. p. 195—205°, obtained from the *Shinchiku* oils Nos. 4, 6 and 10, were subjected to oxidation with Beckmann's chromic acid mixture, and the reaction-product was subsequently treated with sodium bisulphite. Then, the usual method for the formation of α-citryl-β-naphtocinchonic acid was applied to the oil which had been isolated by the decomposition of the bisulphite compound with soda. As a result of this experiment, an acid was obtained, which melted at 195° after repeated crystallisation. Owing to the presence of adherent impurities, attempts to separate the acid in a still purer form have so far led to no result.

(6) Terpinenol - 4.

Despite repeated fractionation of fraction IV, the larger proportion of the distillate boiling between 207 and 213° remained almost unchanged in bulk. The following tests were made with the main fractions possessing the constants :—

B. p. 208—210°, $d_{11°}$ 0·9415, $a_{D11°}$+ 24·50°.

" 210—212°, " 0·948, " + 24·30°.

(A) Formation of terpinene terpin.

By treating these distillates with 5% solution of sulphuric acid a good yield was obtained of terpinene terpin, m. p. 137°; hence, the presence of terpinenol-4 in the oil is presumable. But since terpinene terpin can also be obtained from sabinene, oxidation with permanganate was introduced in the test as the most reliable method.

(B) Formation of 1·2·4·trihydroxyterpane.

30 g. of the fraction under examination were shaken up mechanically with a mixture of 100 g. $KMnO_4$, 42 g. KOH, 2800 g. ice and 2200 g. H_2O. Having observed the satisfactory effect of oxidation, it was further treated in the familiar manner. After filtration, the liquid was evaporated in a current of carbon dioxide gas to about 200 cc. By agitating this evaporated residue in the warm state with chloroform, which is a suitable solvent, a glycerol could easily be extracted in a yield of about 50% of the oil used. The glycerol, after being

purified once or twice from the same solvent, showed a m. p. of from
112 to 114°, which, when repeatedly crystallised, rose to 116—117°.
This body is not bitter in taste and is freely soluble in water and
alcohols; when carefully heated, it sublimes in lustrous crystals melting
at 126—129°. The analysis gave the following figures :—

$$0·1240 \text{ g. subst.}: \quad 0·2896 \text{ g. } CO_2, \; 0·1170 \text{ g. } H_2O.$$

	Found :	Calc. for $C_{10} H_{17} (OH)_3$:
C	63·69%	63·83%
H	10·48%	10·63%.

Although it was evident from the above that the glycerol is
unquestionably 1 · 2 · 4 - trihydroxyterpane, the following experiments
were made to confirm it more definitely.

I. Oxidation of the glycerol with alkaline permanganate solution.

On oxidation with diluted permanganate solution in the presence
of alkali, under cooling, the glycerol yielded, as the resultant product,
$a \cdot a'$ - dihydroxy - a - methyl - a' - isopropyl adipic acid with a m. p. of
205°. It was also observed in another experiment that the acid began
to soften slightly at 188°, trickled at about 192°, and melted completely
at 202° with indications suggesting the presence of the corresponding
inactive acid. When heated by itself or boiled with dilute hydrochloric
acid, it was readily converted into a dilactone of the m. p. 69—71°,
volatile with steam, instead of that which melts at 63—64°; and on
further recrystallisation it yielded the dilactone with m. p. 72—73°,
which, according to Prof. Wallach, is a derivative of the inactive acid.
Hence the simultaneous existence of the two dilactones may be assumed.

Moreover, this dihydroxy-acid could readily be resolved into
ω - dimethyl acetonyl acetone by oxidising it with permanganate in dilute

sulphuric acid solution. ω-dimethyl acetonyl acetone thus obtained was identified by its semicarbazone, m. p. 199—201°.

II. Splitting up of the glycerol into cymene and carvenone.

When the glycerol was boiled with dilute hydrochloric acid, the solution very quickly became turbid, water being eliminated, and there resulted a mixture of p-cymene and carvenone. As a means of identification of carvenone thus formed, the oil-portion was steam-distilled, and by reacting with semicarbazid upon the last-distilled portion in the usual manner, a-carvenone semicarbazone, melting at about 200°, was readily obtained.

The glycerol was also subjected to oxidation with chromic acid anhydride, but attempts to detect ketolactone of the m. p. 63°, which is derived from $1 \cdot 2 \cdot 8$-trioxymenthane, were unsuccessful.

III. Optical rotation of the glycerol.

In comparing the glycerol obtained from *Shô-Gyū* oil with those already known, it is found to bear a close resemblance to the latter, as shown in the following table :—

Glycerols	Specific rotation of 1·2·4-trioxyterpane	Solvent	p	t°
Glycerol obtained from terpinenol-4 of Ceylon cardamom oil	+21·24°	Ethyl alcohol	9·6	22°
That obtained from terpinenol-4 of marjoram oil	+20·62°	"	10·17	23°
That obtained from terpinenol-4 produced by treating sabinene with sulphuric acid	+21·21°	"	10·84	—
That obtained from terpinenol-4 contained in our *Shô-Gyū* oil	+21·27°	."	10·19	20°

From the above data, it is to be concluded that terpinenol - 4 occurs to a considerable extent in the original oil, inasmuch as the glycerol has been proved to be identical with $1 \cdot 2 \cdot 4$ - trihydroxyterpane. At the same time, the reason why the specific gravity of the fraction under examination is slightly higher than that of terpinenol - 4 will be seen by observing the fact that piperonylic acid of the m. p. $227°$ was obtained, although in small quantity, from the mother liquor, out of which the glycerol had been removed after the permanganate oxidation of the test oil.

On different occasion, for the purpose of obtaining crystallising derivatives from the terpinenol oil-portion, the fraction that boiled between $205°$ and $217°$, constituting nearly ¾ of fraction IV, was fractionated repeatedly *in vacuo*, and finally distilled at ordinary pressure. The main portion, boiling, at $208 \cdot 5—211°$, was split up into several portions, which were found to possess the following constants :—

I	B.p. 207 —208·5°	$d_{8°}$ 0·939	$\alpha_{D8°} + 25 \cdot 00°$	$n_{D18°}$ 1·47743
2	// 208·5—209°	// 0·941	// $+ 25 \cdot 80°$	// 1·47812
3	// 209 —209·5°	// 0·944	// $+ 26 \cdot 30°$	// 1·47812*
4	// 209·5—211°	// 0·949	// $+ 26 \cdot 08°$	// 1·48007

From these fractions solid derivatives could be obtained as desired.

* This fraction, when oxidised with permanganate, also produced the glycerol, m.p. 111—114°, the yield of which was about 95% of the material employed. When warmed up with twice its quantity of pure formic acid, terpinene was formed, water being eliminated. The crude terpinene thus obtained possessed the following constants: b. p. 175—185°, $d_{27°}$ 0·850, $\alpha_{D25°} + 0·87°$, $n_{D25°}$ 1·47635, and, when further oxidised with diluted permanganate solution in the cold, yielded erythritol, m. p. 237—238°, together with i-α·α'-dihydroxy-α-methyl-α'-isopropyladipic acid, m. p. 188—189°.

1) Nitrosochloride. By the action of amyl nitrite and hydrochloric acid in a solution of glacial acetic acid, all the fractions gave a nitrosochloride, the yield of which was about 20—25% of the material used. When twice recrystallised from acetic ester, it showed the m. p. 111—112°. The chlorine determination and the result of combustion gave the following figures which agree with those theoretically required :

 I. 0·2337 g. subst. :   0·4708 g. CO_2, 0·1782 g. H_2O.

 II. 0·4377 g.   0·2819 g. AgCl.

   Found :   Calc. for $C_{10}H_{17}$ (OH) NOCl :

  C 54·94%   54·67%

  H 8·47%   8·20%

  Cl 15·93%   16·17%.

2) Nitrolpiperidide. When treated with alcoholic piperidine as usual, the nitrosochloride was readily converted into its nitrolpiperidide. In spite of the purity of the preparation, the m. p. could not be fixed at the first stage. After repeated recrystallisation from methyl alcohol, however, it was obtained in the pure state and melted at 172—174°. The nitrolpiperidide differs from that of a-terpineol by the m. p. and crystal form, while the corresponding nitrosochloride has nearly the same m. p. Combustion gave the following satisfactory result :—

  0·2142 g. subst. :   0·5244 g. CO_2, 0·2023 g. H_2O.

   Found :   Calc. for $C_{10}H_{17}$ (OH) $NONC_5H_{10}$:

  C 66·77%   67·16%

  H 10·49%   10·45%.

3) Phenylurethane. When mixed with phenyl isocyanate and left to stand for at least a fortnight, the terpinenol fractions congealed into solid crystalline mass, from which a phenylurethane could be obtained quantitatively. The solidification of the reaction-mixture may be accelerated by inoculation with small crystals of the pure urethane. Recrystallised from light petroleum ether, which is the most suitable solvent, it crystallises out in long needles, and melts at 71—72°.

The alcoholic solution of this body shows a rotation to the right as docs the original fraction itself.

Combustion :—

I. 0.2883 g. subst. :   0.7930 g. CO_2, 0.2250 g. H_2O.

II. 0.3162 g.   //   0.8674 g. // 0.2445 g. //

Found :   Calc. for $C_6 H_5 NHCOOC_{10} H_{17}$:

	I.	II.	
C	75.01%	74.81%	74.72%
H	8.66%	8.56%	8.42%.

4) **Naphtylurethane.** With a - naphtyl isocyanate, the terpinenol fractions also formed a solid derivative at the end of two weeks. The compound crystallises from its alcoholic solution in white needles and when purified by means of dilute methyl alcohol melts at 105·5—106·5°.

Upon combustion it gave the following figures :—

0·2077 g. subst. :   0·5902 g. CO_2, 0·1536 g. H_2O.

	Found :	Calc. for $C_{21} H_{25} NO_2$:
C	77·50%	78·02%
H	8·21%	8·74%.

From what has been stated above, the conclusion may be drawn that the terpinenol contained in our *Shô-Gyū* oil produces not only urethanes but a nitrosochloride as well. Furthermore, in order to investigate the question whether the last-named body can actually be derived from the terpinenol, the following manipulation was pursued.

The phenylurethane which can be prepared without difficulty in the pure state was split up by boiling it for 4—5 hours with alcoholic potash. After the elimination of the solvent the resulting oil-portion was liberated by means of water and shaken with tartaric acid solution to remove aniline that had been formed in the process of decomposition of the urethane. The crude alcohol prepared in this manner, after being purified by distillation with steam, boiled at 207—209°. Treated with nitrosyl chloride, this alcohol yielded a nitrosochloride (m. p. 112—113°) of which the corresponding nitrolpiperidide (impure) had a m. p. of from 165 to 168°; when oxidised with permanganate in the cold it reverted into 1·2·4-trihydroxyterpane, m. p. 111—114°. Owing to the scarcity of material available it was impossible further to investigate the problem.

The examination concerning this alcohol-fraction together with heavy oil-portions is being continued.

———————

Camphor. Examination having failed to detect camphor in oil No. 1, fraction III was submitted to repeated fractionation, and the resulting distillate boiling between 250—215° was tested for the formation of oxim according to Angeli and Rimini's method; but the result was negative. On the other hand, the fraction (b. p. 205—208°) of oil No. 8, which had been proved to contain a large proportion of heavy oil, when examined for the presence of camphor by the same method, yielded only a very small quantity of a brownish oil.

Repeated attempts to find *a-terpineol* (the presence of which appeared to be probable) from the fraction boiling between 215 and 225° of oil No. 1 were also without result.

(7) Geraniol.

Fraction V was fractionally distilled under reduced pressure, and the distillate boiling between 97—112° (8 mm.), after having been shaken with 5% caustic soda liquor in order to remove phenolic substances, was again distilled. The result of distillation was as follows :—

B. p. 101°   (8 mm.), $d_{7°}$ 0·985, $a_{D7°}$ +17·50°.
  //   101—105° //   ,   // 1·017,   // +11·30°.

Adding 50 parts of phthalic anhydride and 100 parts of benzene to 100 parts of the test-liquid, the mixture was warmed for three hours in a water-bath at 80° ; then the method for isolating acid phthalic ester was pursued as usual. On subsequent saponification, an oil with a geraniol-like odour was obtained as the product ; hence, (1) the formation of citral on oxidation with chromic acid, and (2) the preparation of diphenyl urethane by Erdmann's method were successively tried. In the former case, there was some indication of the presence of citral from its odour, whereas in the latter, which is known as the simplest and most reliable test, it failed to form the generally well-crystallising diphenyl urethane. Since geraniol appeared, from these tests, to occur in oil No. 1 in a very small proportion, oil No. 8 was subsequently examined. Adding 100 g. of phthalic anhydride to 250 g. of the fraction of oil No. 8, with the constants : b.p. 99—101° (7 mm.), $d_{5°}$ 1·045, $a_{D5°}$ +7·20°, the mixture was heated in a water-bath for three hours, and the product of reaction was then further treated in the familiar manner. The resulting oil-portion which was liberated by saponification with alcoholic potash, when purified by steam-distillation, developed a well-defined odour of rose, but the quantity of this body was so small that the yield amounted to only

0·04% of the original oil. To proceed still further in the test, 2·5 cc. of the oil together with the definite proportions of pyridine and diphenyl carbamine chloride was treated in the usual manner. From this reaction-product, a compound was readily obtained, which in the crude state melted at 62—63°, and after purification showed the m. p. 80·5°. Judging from (1) its needle-shaped crystals, and (2) the yellow coloration with concentrated sulphuric acid, which changes into indigo-blue after the addition of nitric acid, this substance was positively confirmed to be geranyl diphenyl urethane. Thus the existence of geraniol was proved.

(8) Citronellol.

Citronellol, which is known to occur naturally in common with geraniol in several essential oils, was also found in oil No. 8. As a test for its presence, 2 cc. of the remaining oil-portion, which had been used for the examination of geraniol, with an addition of 2 g. of phthalic anhydride, were heated in a water-bath for two hours. The product of reaction was further purified by rinsing several times with boiling water. Then, the silver salt was prepared according to Erdmann's direction. By fractional crystallisation from benzene and methyl alcohol, two silver salts could be isolated from it. Of these, one produced first, which melted distinctly at 133°, was confirmed to be the silver salt of geraniol phthalic ester acid, and the other, obtained later, which had m. p. 125—126°, to be that of citronellol phthalic ester acid. The presence of citronellol is therefore presumable.

(9) Safrol.

Safrol is found to a considerable extent in the heavy oil-portion of *Shô-Gyū* oil, and is easily detected as in the case of heavy camphor or *Shiu* oil. Its presence, for instance, in the fraction (d_4. 1·013, $a_{D4°}$ +12·70°) obtained from fraction V, was also presumable from the odour and specific gravity. To submit it to a further test, the distillate was shaken together with 5% caustic soda liquor in order to remove phenolic ingredients, and, after distillation, a fraction distilling between 225 and 235° was oxidised with potassium permanganate, when, as the last oxidised product of safrol, piperonylic acid melting at 228° was obtained ; thus easily proving the presence of safrol. Among the distillates of oil No. 8, the remaining fraction, which passed over above 221°, with the constants: $d_{21°}$ 1·052, $a_{D21°}$ +4·00°, was heated with alcoholic potash in order to convert the allyl-group into the propenyl-group, and was afterwards oxidised with chromic acid, thereby piperonal of the m. p. 37° being readily obtained (m. p. of the semicarbazone 225°). Hence the presence of safrol in oil No. 8 was easily determined ; besides, its existence in the *Shinchiku* oils Nos. 4, 7, and 9 was similarly confirmed.

(10) Eugenol.

The isolation of this substance, which occurs with safrol in many essential oils, was ,readily accomplished by shaking the safrol fraction (for example, the remaining distillate of oil No. 8 : d_8. 1·045, $a_{D6°}$ +8·75°) with a 5% caustic soda solution. After being liberated from the alkaline aqueous solution, the crude eugenol oil-portion was purified by steam-distillation. When treated with benzoyl chloride according to Schotten - Baumann's method, it yielded benzoyl eugenol, melting at 69°, thus proving the presence of eugenol in the oil.

Cadinene. . The quantity of residue over the boiling point of eugenol obtained from *Shinchiku* oils Nos. 1 and 8 being very small, only the colour reaction of cadinene was tested. When the sesquiterpene fraction dissolved in glacial acetic acid was treated with concentrated sulphuric acid as usual, a deep-green colour appeared, which first changed into indigo-blue, and then into purplish-red. Consequently, the presence of this sesquiterpene may be presumed.

———————

From the concise descriptions of various experiments made thus far, a general knowledge of the composition of *Shô-Gyū* oil may be had. The existence of sabinene, dipentene, a - as well as γ - terpinene, terpinenol - 4, citronellol, geraniol, safrol and eugenol has been definitely ascertained, while that of formaldehyde, linalool and cadinene may be presumed from their colour reaction. Thus it appears that *Shô-Gyū* oil resembles Ceylon cardamom oil in the presence of sabinene, terpinene and terpinenol - 4, and its odour recalls sweet marjoram oil ; besides, it possesses numerous features common to savin, nutmeg, and even juniper oil. An oil with these properties and the prospects of yielding several hundred thousand *kin* per annum, duly deserves public recognition as one of the chief essential oils produced in Formosa.

—————◼◆◼—————

PART II

Investigation of the Essential Oil
of *Yu-Ju*

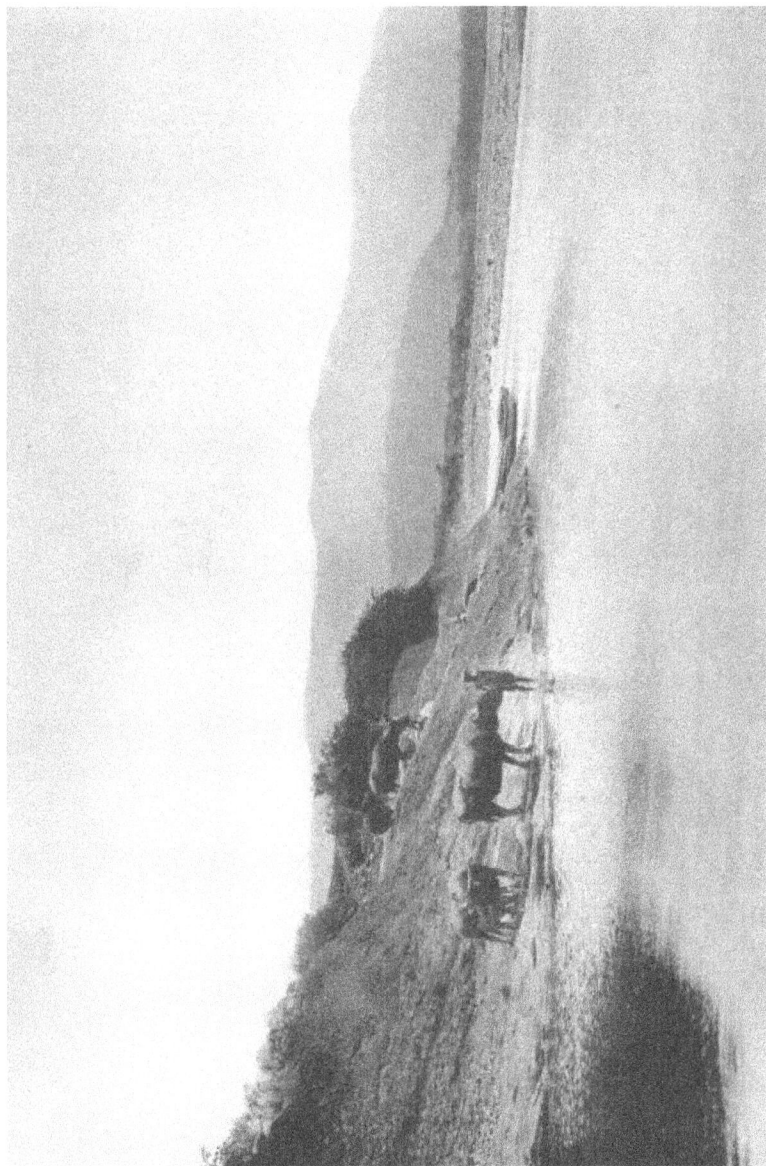

The *Nawasen-kei* as seen from *Punkiko* on the *Kōsempo* road.

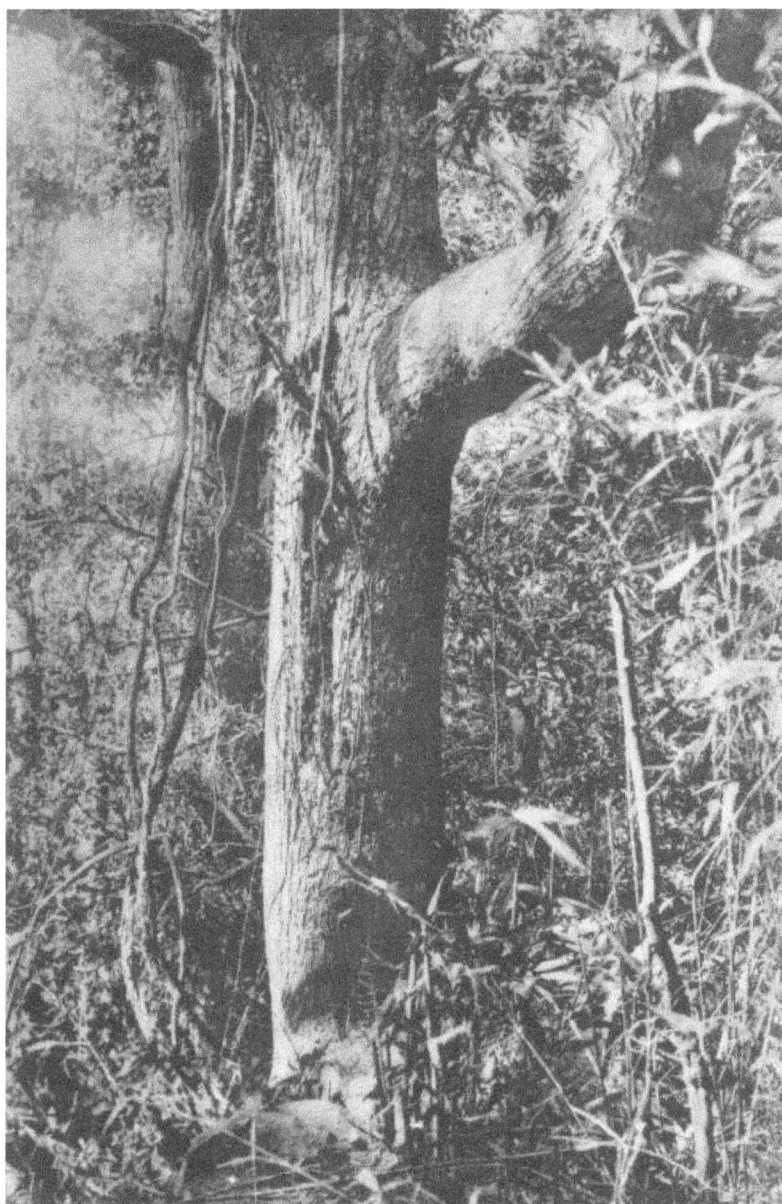

Yu-fu tree in *Shinkôkô*.

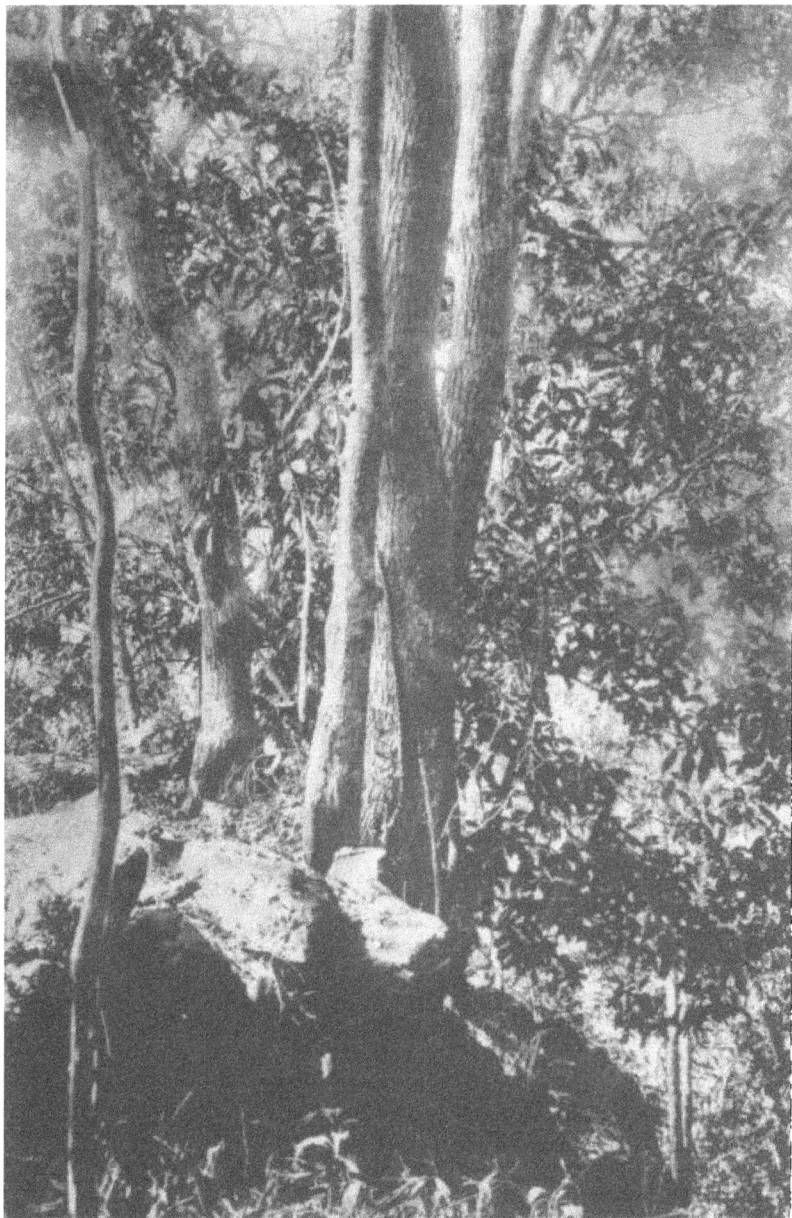

Yu-Ju trees on summit of Mount *Shinkōkō*.

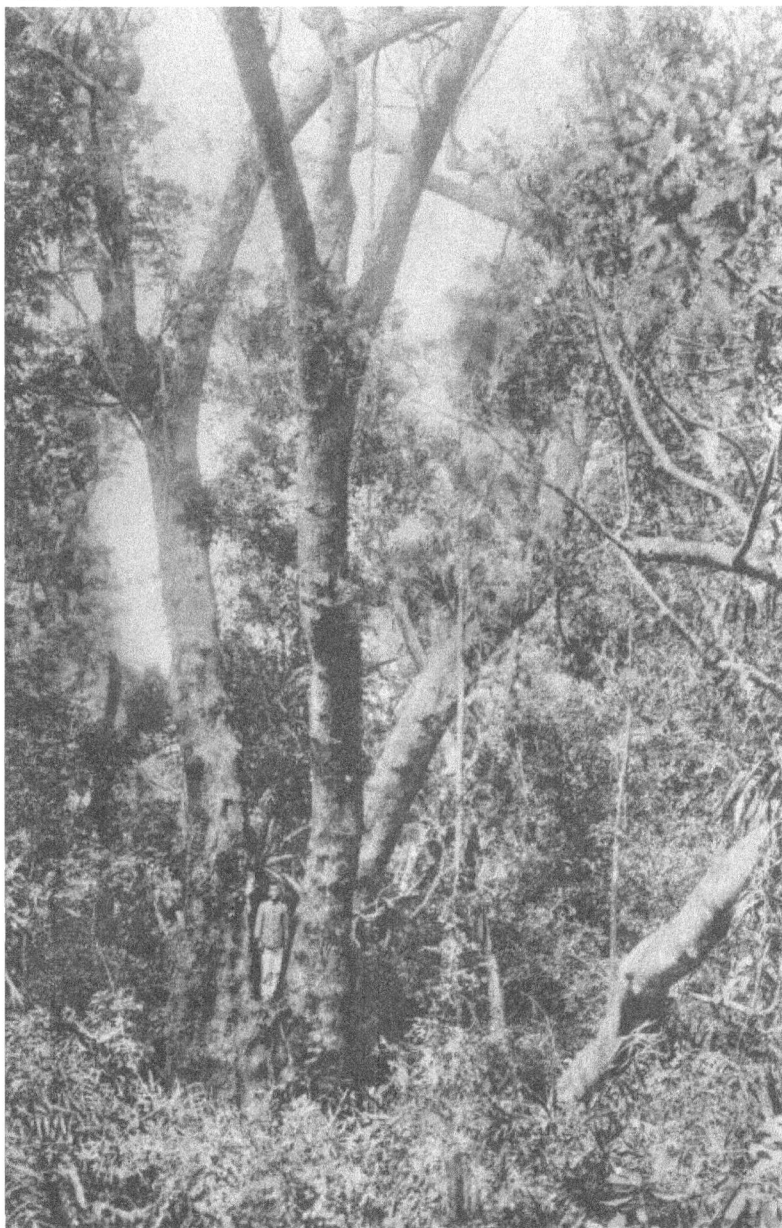

A huge *Yu-Ju* tree near Camphor Distillery No. 5.

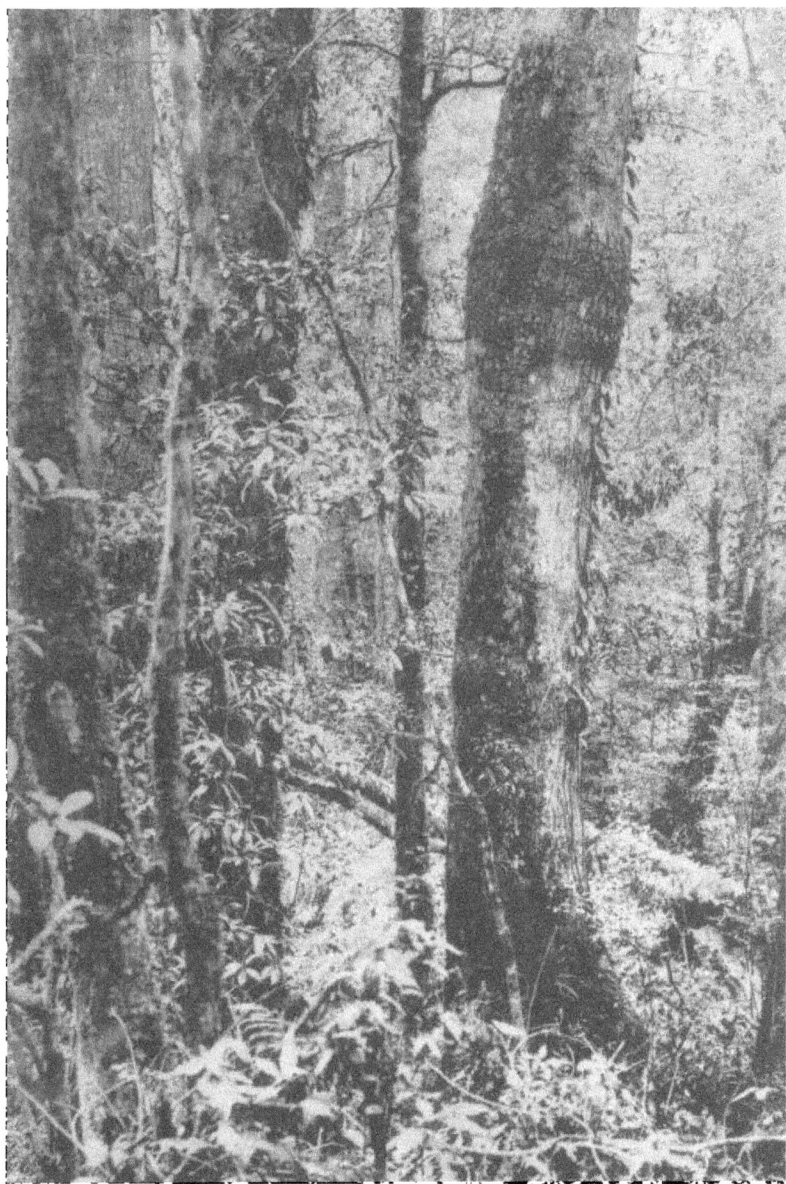

Yu-Ju forest in vicinity of *Shinkôkô*.

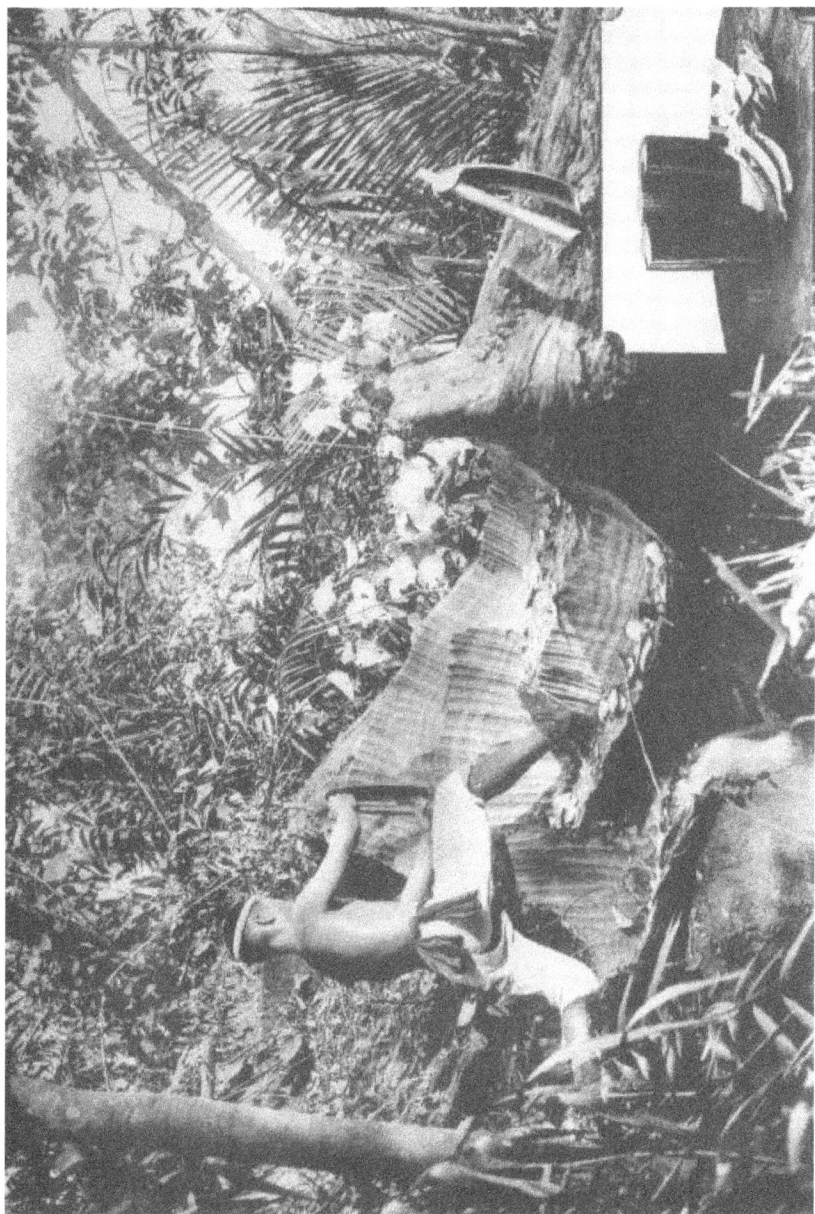

Chopping *Ju-Ju* wood.

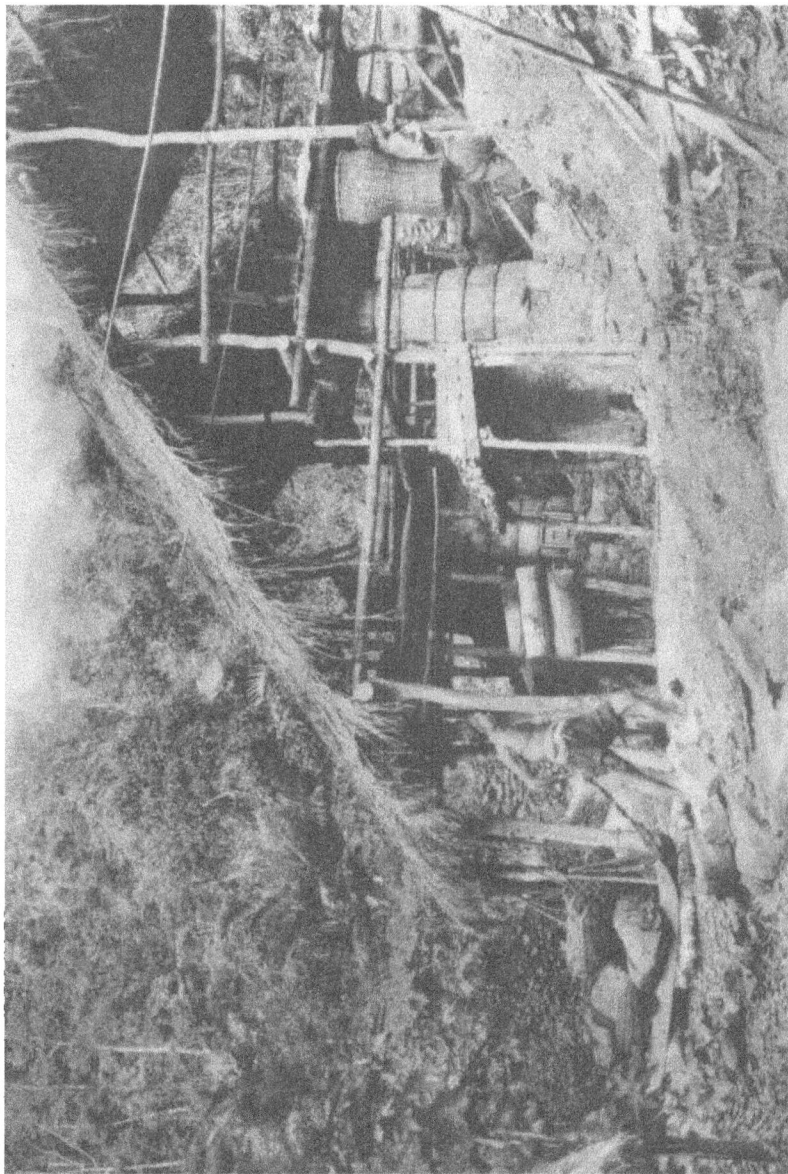

Full view of Camphor Distillery No. 5, *Shinkōkō*.

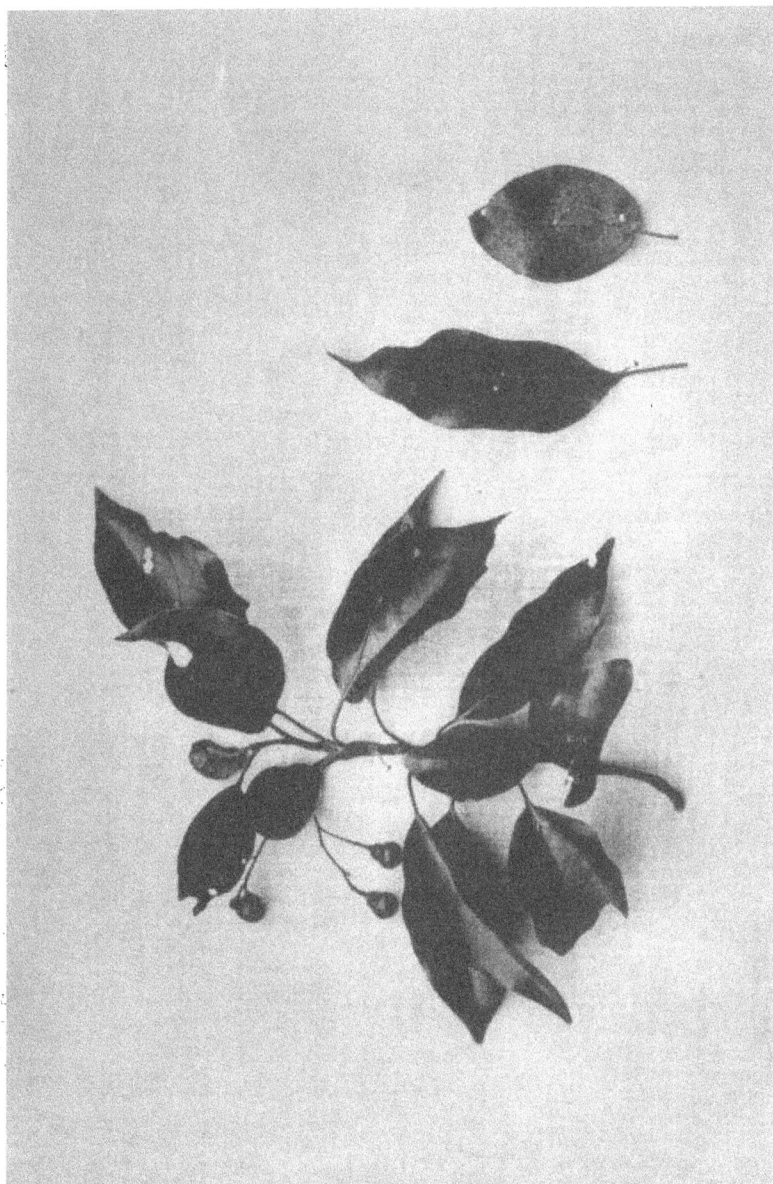

Leaves and fruit of *Ya-Ju* tree in *Kösempö*.

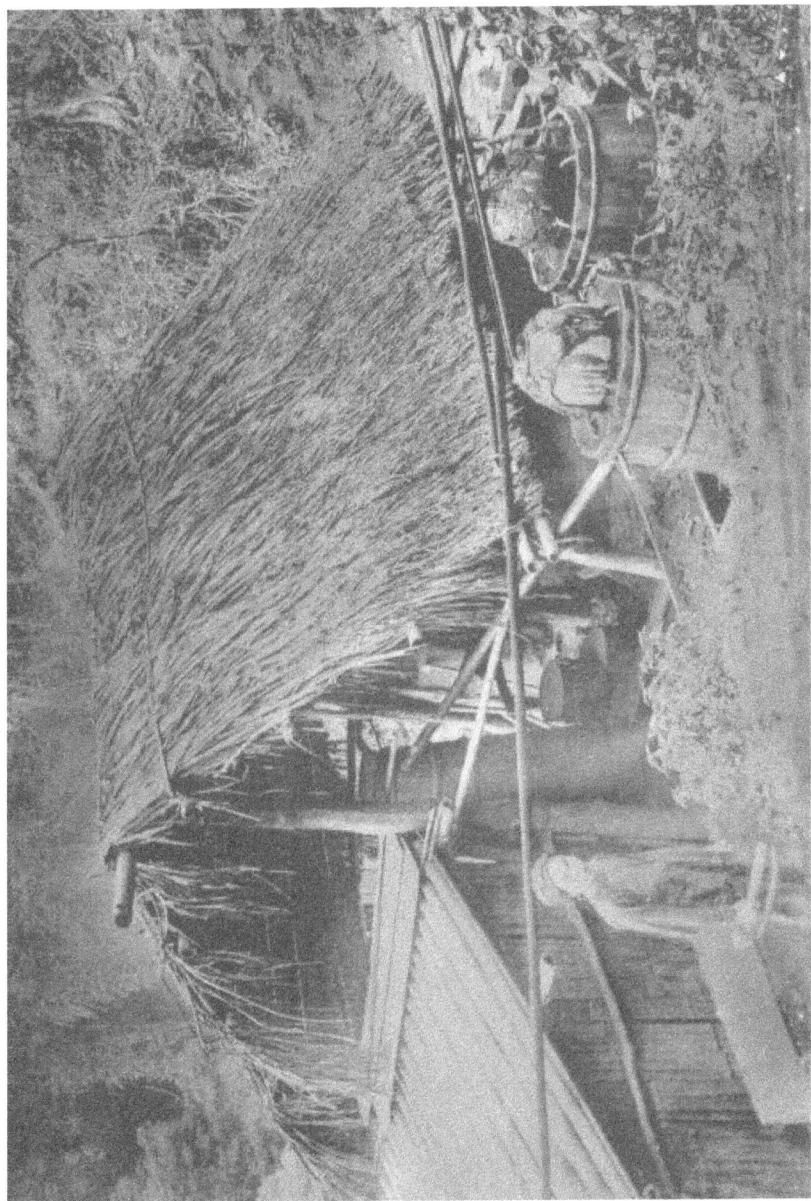

The "*Kame*" system of distillation (Camphor Distillery No. 111, *Tovôyen*).

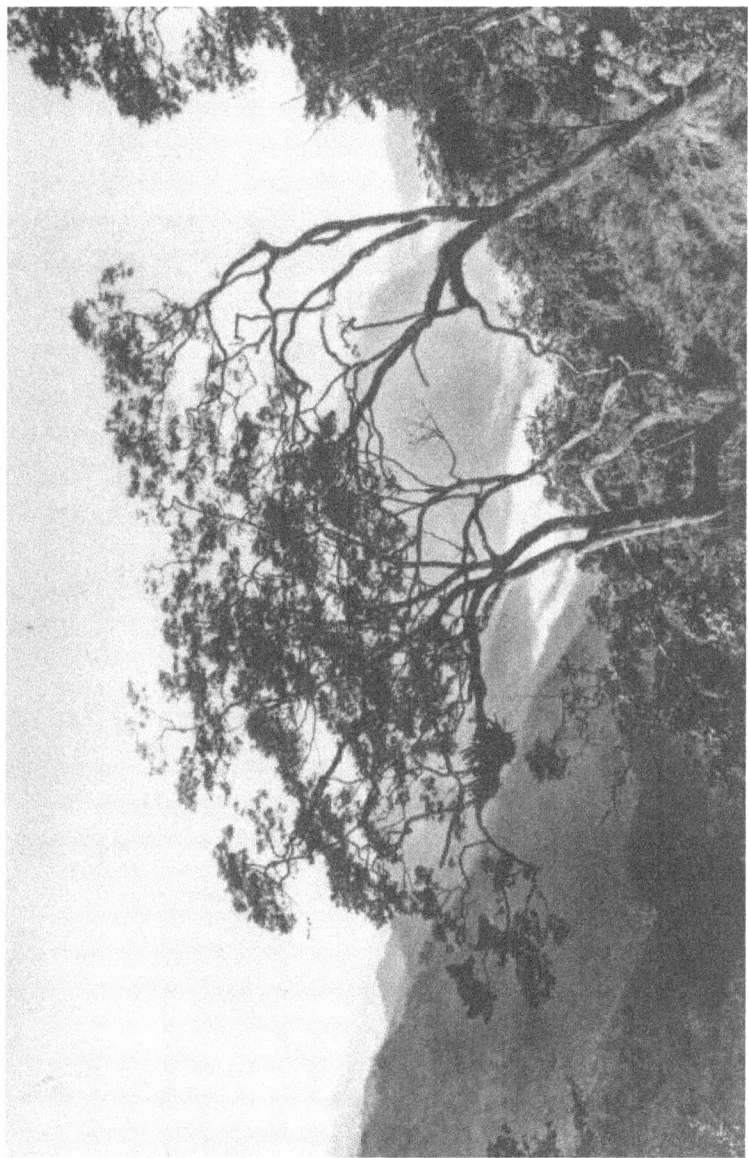

Camphor trees in *Arisan*.

CONTENTS.

	PAGE
Yu-Ju Oil and *Yu-Ju* ··· ··· ··· ··· ··· ··· ··· ··· ··· ··· ···	1
Location of the *Yu-Ju* Districts ··· ··· ··· ··· ··· ··· ··· ··· ···	1
Yield and Total Production of *Yu-Ju* Oil ··· ··· ··· ··· ··· ···	2
Physical Properties of *Yu-Ju* Oil ··· ··· ··· ··· ··· ··· ··· ···	3
Examination of *Yu-Ju* Oil by Distillation ··· ··· ··· ··· ··· ···	4
Constituents of *Yu-Ju* Oil ··· ··· ··· ··· ··· ··· ··· ··· ··· ···	8
I. The Hydrocarbon Fraction ··· ··· ··· ··· ··· ··· ···	8
II. The Camphor Fraction ··· ··· ··· ··· ··· ··· ··· ···	11
III. The Safrol Fraction ··· ··· ··· ··· ··· ··· ··· ··· ···	12

Yu-Ju Oil and Yu-Ju.

" Yu-Ju oil " is a term applied to an essential oil which is obtained from the so-called " Oil Tree ", indigenous to southern Formosa, and which is closely related to camphor oil in its properties. Its failure, however, to yield camphor in the course of production is the chief feature differing from camphor oil, and evidently indicates the reason why the natives call the mother-tree, " Iû-chhiu "* or " Oil Tree ". Similarly, the term " Yu-bôku " or " Yu-bun-bôku ",† as frequently applied by the Japanese to the tree, which yields only a little camphor and a large quantity of oil, suggests the inconspicuously small percentage of camphor obtainable.

The Yu-Ju tree is identical, in its external forms, with the camphor tree (Cinnamomum Camphora, NEES et EBERM.), and the camphor-manufacturers mainly rely, as the sole means of discriminating between them, upon the odour of shavings taken from the root, outside of which no particular method seems to be in current use.

Location of the Yu-Ju Districts.

Since the camphor-tree growing in southern Formosa generally yields, as stated in the preface, a small quantity of camphor and a copious amount of oil, it may be designated, in a comprehensive way, the " Yu-Ju-camphor-tree ". In addition to Karenkô (Hoe-lieng-kang) and Daitô (Tai-tang) prefectures, which possess vast growing tracts, Kagi

---

* Yu or Iû (油) = oil; Ju or Chhiu (樹) = tree.

† Yu bun = oil portion ; bôku = tree.

prefecture embraces also such a district as *Tanhaiku* bordering *Kōsempo*, where the tree commonly yields six times as much oil as camphor; thus giving a fair notion of the extent to which the tree is flourishing even in this prefecture. *Akō* prefecture also figures prominently as one of the leading producing centres, *Rônô-kei* (*Lau-lông-khoe*), *Dakkô-kei* (*Lôk-hau-khoe*), and the entire tract stretching along the *Namasen-kei* being the main districts.

According to the statement of a member of the *Kōsempo* Camphor Distillery, the comparative outputs of camphor and the oil portion are at the average proportion of 25 to 75, showing that an enormous amount of the oil is producible. In *Banshoryô* (*Han-chû-liâu*), *Shinkôkô* (*Chhim-kau-kiⁿ*), *Daipanriau* (*Lai-pang-liâu*) and *Datetsu* (*Phah-thih*), celebrated as the chief *Yu-Ju* growing localities, some varieties often totally fail to yield stearoptene, the average yield of which generally is not more than ten percent of the oil-portion produced.

Yield and Total Production of *Yu-Ju* Oil.

The *Yu-Ju* oil is readily obtained, as in the case of ordinary camphor oil, by the prevalent *Tosa* system. According to the investigation carried out by a member of the *Kōsempo* Camphor Distilley, the maximum yield of camphor oil obtained from a *Yu-Ju*-camphor-tree in that district is 5%, and a yield of 4% is considered to be fairly excellent, while the figure occasionally falls to the minimum of 1%. But an average yield of 2% may be reasonably regarded as a standard.

In comparison with the *Kōsempo* camphor oil just mentioned, the real *Yu-Ju* oil, being considered more copious in its yield, may also be safely estimated at 3 to 4%. Despite the fact that the existing stocks of the *Yu-Ju* tree are much fewer than those of the *Yu-Ju*-camphor-tree, and that no large amount of production could be expected, an output of 50,000 to 60,000 *kin* per annum would not be a matter of difficulty.

Physical Properties of *Yu-Ju* Oil.

The *Yu-Ju* oil is identical with camphor oil in physical properties except in optical activity, in which the former seems to be slightly weaker. Usually, it has a light yellow or golden or, very rarely, a greenish-yellow, colour, but certain varieties of camphor oil produced from the *Yu-Ju*-camphor-tree growing in *Kōsempo*, frequently possess, as exceptions, an intense brown colour, or are altogether devoid of colour.

The specific gravity and optical rotation of the different varieties of the oil may be gleaned from the following table.

Place of origin	No.	Colour	d at t°		a_D at t°		n_D at t°	
Shinkôkô	1	Light golden yellow	0·945	13	+ 29·22°	13	1·47596	19
"	2	"	0·942	"	+ 18·88°	"	1·47457	"
"	3	"	0·951	12	+ 19·50°	12	1·47869	20
"	4	"	0·967	13½	+ 22·48°	13½	1·48191	19
"	5	"	0·966	"	+ 24·42°	"	1·48568	20
"	6	Golden yellow	0·961	14	+ 29·85°	14	1·48045	20½
"	7	"	0·961	"	+ 26·52°	"	1·48326	21
"	8	Light golden yellow	0·963	15	+ 26·95°	15	1·48326	"
"	9	Golden yellow	0·955	"	+ 25·35°	"	1·47850	20
"	10	Light golden yellow	0·947	"	+ 27·30°	"	1·47567	19½
Daipanriau	11 (a)	Slightly greenish yellow	0·954	16	+ 21·00°	16	1·47694	19
"	11 (b)	"	0·953	"	+ 21·30°	"	1·47694	"
"	12 (a)	"	0·972	"	+ 30·80°	"	1·47746	"
"	12 (b)	Light golden yellow	0·951	"	+ 28·30°	"	1·48278	"

The oil is easily distinguished from *Shiu* oil by the absence of the linalool colour-reaction with mercuric sulphate.

Examination of *Yu-Ju* Oil by Distillation.

TABLE SHOWING THE RESULTS OF FRACTIONAL DISTILLATION
OF *YU-JU* OIL.

No. 1. No. 2.

B. p.	%	d at t°	α_D at t°	Mother liquid freed from camphor by filtration			%	d at t°	α_D at t°	Mother liquid freed from camphor by filtration		
				%	$d_{t°}$	$α_{Dt°}$				%	$d_{t°}$	$α_{Dt°}$
Up to 180°	7·00	0·900 14	+22·64 14				14·00	0·900 18	+13·25 18			
180—185°	} 23·75	0·908 "	+24·64 "				25·50	0·904 "	+14·70 "			
185—190°							8·00	0·918 "	+17·70 "			
190—195°	11·25	0·926 "	+28·00 "				8·50	0·927 19	+20·33 "			
195—200°	7·70	0·940 15	+30·53 15				8·20	0·939 "	+22·65 "			
200—205°	} 18·5?						10·00					
205—210°												
210—217°				23·20_22	0·977_18	+25·70_16	15·50			22·9O_16	0·977_18	+23·30_18
217—218°	} 17·50											
218—220°												
Residue	9·30	0·997 "	?				10·30	1·000 "	?			

No. 3. No. 4.

B. p.	%	d at t°	α_D at t°	Mother liquid			%	d at t°	α_D at t°	Mother liquid		
Up to 180°	10·50	0·900 19	+14·35 19				} 6·50	0·908 18	+17·25 18			
180—185°	13·50	0·904 19½	+15·25 19½									
185—190°	7·00	0·913 19	+17·30 19				14·50	0·914 "	+19·00 "			
190—195°	9·75	0·925 "	+19·45 "				12·40	0·925 "	+21·69 "			
195—200°	8·25	0·937 "	+22·60 "				9·75	0·939 "	+24·65 "			
200—205°	7·25	0·950 "	+23·75 "				6·50	0·954 "	+27·40 "			
205—210°	7·50			16·75_18	0·979_18	+23·50_18	8·00			23·00_18	0·991_18	+24·75_18
210—217°	11·75						19·50					
217—218°	} 7·00	0·998 "	+20·25 18				} 6·40	1·006 "	+22·20 "			
218—220°												
Residue	17·50	1·006 "	?				16·45	1·026 "	?			

No. 5.

Range				
Up to 180° / 180—185°	16·50	0·896 18	+23·35	18
185—190°	12·90	0·904 //	+24·93	//
190—195°	9·40	0·917 //	+26·82	//
195—200° / 200—205°	9·00	0·935 //	+28·72	//
205—210°	7·75	0·965 //	+29·75	//
210—217°	16 00			
217—218°	2·75			
218—220°	6·00	1·004 //	+23·83	//
Residue	19·70	1·027 //	+17·20	//

Brace: 16·90_{18}, 0·993_{18}, +26·75_{18}

No. 6.

Range				
Up to 180° / 180—185°	6·75	0·897 22	+25·75	22
185—190°	9·00	0·905 //	+27·64	//
190—195°	11·65	0·920 //	+31·00	//
195—200°	13·00	0·934 //	+33·16	//
200—205°	18·00			
205—210°				
210—217°	24·50			
217—218° / 218—220°	5·00	1·002 //	+26·06	//
Residue	12·10	1·012 //	+18·60	//

Brace: 27·50_{20}, 0·980_{20}, +28·25_{20}

No. 7.

Range				
Up to 180°	5·00	0·894 22	+26·00	22
180—185°	6·20	0.893 21	+26·14	21
185—190°	12·00	c 905 //	+28·40	//
190—195°	10·00	0·916 21½	+29·98	21½
195—200°	8·20	0·930 //	+31·36	//
200—205°	6·35	0·949 //	+32·50	//
205—210°	8·65			
210—217°	19·50			
217—218° / 218—220°	5·75	1·003 //	+24·50	//
Residue	18·35	1·015 //	+17·25	//

Brace: 23·00_{21}, 0·988_{18}, +27·97_{18}

No. 8.

Range				
Up to 180° / 180—185°	9·25	0·898 22	+24·56	22
185—190°	14·00	0·907 //	+26·45	//
190—195°	8·75	0·920 //	+29·00	//
195—200°	5·25	—	+30·80	//
200—205° / 205—210°	19·45			
210—217°	19·30			
217—218° / 218—220°	5·90	1·004 //	+25·00	//
Residue	18·10	1·018 //	+18·45	//

Brace: 32·35_{21}, 0·976_{21}, +28·50_{21}

No. 9. No. 10.

	No. 9								No. 10							
Up to 180° / 180—185°	9·55	0·904	23	+20·16	23				19·25	0·901	23	+21·75	23			
185—190°	13·40	0·911	//	+22·00	//				11·75	0·909	22	+24·00	22			
190—195°	11·50	0·922	//	+24·35	//				6·75	0·921	//	+27·36	//			
195—200°	11·10	0·935	//	+27·30	//				8·00	0·933	23	+29·96	23	7·95$_{23}$		
200—205° / 205—210°	15·90								26·00							
210—217°	19·00					32·00$_{22}$	0·975$_{22}$	+23·64$_{22}$	14·50					27·50$_{25}$	0·964$_{23}$	+25·50$_{23}$
217—218° / 218—220°	4·25								2·00							
Residue	15·30	0·998	//	+21·30	//				11·75	0·992	//	?				

No. 11 (a). No. 11 (b).

	No. 11 (a)								No. 11 (b)							
Up to 180°	8·50	0·903	22	+15·40	22				7·65	0·900	22	+15·30	22			
180—185°	10·50	0·905	21	+16·00	21				9·75	0·905	//	+16·50	//			
185—190°	14·00	0·915	//	+18·43	//				14·50	0·914	//	+19·69	//			
190—195°	11·50	0·930	//	+21·25	//				10·00	0·925	//	+20·75	//			
195—200°	7·20	0·941	//	+24·40	//				11·05	0·941	//	+24·40	//			
200—205° / 205—210°	16·75								14·20							
210—217°						34·70$_{22}$	0·975$_{21}$	+23·50$_{21}$	17·25					25·50$_{22}$	0·973$_{22}$	+23·50$_{22}$
217—218° / 218—220°	22·50								5·65	0·996	//	+20·90	//			
Residue	9·05	1·014	//	?					9·95	1·013	//	?				

No. 12 (a). No. 12 (b).

	No. 12 (a)								No. 12 (b)								
Up to 180°	9·10	0·896	21	+24·65	21												
180—185°	14·75	0·900	//	+25·25	//				12·85	0·911	21	+26·25	21				
185—190°	8·30	0·914	//	+28·05	//												
190—195°	15·20	0·932	//	+32·25	//				9·25	0·925	22	+28·23	22				
195—200°	.								7·75	0·938	0	+30·65	//				
200—205°	27·50					$29·60_{21}$	$0·981_{21}$	$+28·30_{21}$	23·10					$38·00_{22}$	$0·983_{22}$	$+28·00_{22}$	
205—210°																	
210—217°	9·25								24·10								
217—218°									3·75								
218—220°									3·50	—		—					
Residue	5·90	1·015	//	?					15·70	1·025	//	?					

The estimation of the camphor mother-liquid in the above table was carried out as follows :—

The camphor fraction was, in the first place, filtered off by a suction pump, and the camphor remaining on the filter paper, after being completely separated from the mother-liquid, was rinsed once with water. Then as much as possible of the small oil-portion, filtered together with water, was collected with the aid of a separating funnel, and added to the main portion of the mother-liquid to be measured.

It will be understood from the above that oils Nos. 2, 3, 4, and 5, having a low optical rotation, yield only a small quantity of camphor on fractional distillation, whereas Nos. 1, 6, 10, and 12 produce a considerably larger amount on account of their higher optical rotation.

Constituents of *Yu-Ju* Oil.

In consideration of a comparatively plentiful supply of the material for testing purposes, and of its physical properties, as well as the results of fractional distillation, oil No. 11 (a) was found to be more suitable for examination of the nature of the oil than other varieties. Accordingly, the following experiments were conducted with it.

As a preliminary process, the oil was fractionally distilled under reduced pressure (15 mm.), and split up into three parts.

No.	d at t°		α_D at t°		Fraction	Remarks
I	0·899	23	+ 15·50°	23	Terpene fraction	
II	0·923	14	+ 20·10°	14	"	
III	0·941	13	+ 25·16°	13	"	{ This fraction yielded camphor when cooled
IV	0·965	23	+ 23·75°	23	Camphor fraction	{ Sp. gr. and opt. rot. in this column are those of the mother-liquid freed from camphor by filtration
V	1·015	14	+ 14·90°	14	Safrol fraction	

I. The Hydrocarbon Fraction.

On redistillation of the first distilled water obtained by distilling the first fraction *in vacuo* (18 mm.), a golden yellow heavy oil was separated, which, with a solution of aniline hydrochloride in aniline, or an alcoholic solution of p-toluidine acetate in p-toluidine, gave an intense red coloration. Owing to the exceedingly small quantity available, the identification of this body was out of the question, but, judging from the characteristic colour-reaction, the presence of **furfurol** in the oil may be presumed.

The formation of nitrosochloride (m. p. 107—108°), nitrolpiperidide (m. p. 117—118°) and nitrosopinene (m. p. 131—132°) from the first hydrocarbon fraction possessing the properties : b. p. 155—158°, d_{23° 0·861, a_{D23° +5·00°, n_{D18° 1·46622, confirms the presence of a-**pinene.**

The presence of **camphene** was also proved by testing the following fractions, according to Bertram and Walbaum's hydration process :

B. p. 158—160°, d_{23° 0·863, a_{D23° +4·50°, n_{D18° 1·46653.
  ,, 160—165°, ,, 0·869,   ,,   +3·00°, n_{D19° 1·46691.

The resultant iso-borneol had a m. p. of 209°, and its phenylurethane melted at 138°.

The fractions with the constants : b. p. 160—165°, d_{23° 0·869, a_{D23° +3·00° and b. p. 164—169°, d_{27° 0·877, a_{D27° +2·75°, which still contained camphene, were oxidised with alkaline permanganate solution, when they yielded, as a resulting product, a small quantity of sodium nopinate. The free nopinic acid had m. p. 126—127°, and was lævorotatory. Hence the presence of β-**pinene** was determined.

Fractions II and III consisted mainly of **cineol.** The fraction distilling over between 175 and 180° with the constants : d_{20° 0·890, a_{D20° +3·65° was first of all shaken with 50% resorcin solution, then, the crystalline addition product separated off was removed from the oil, and finally decomposed with the addition of caustic soda liquor.

The cineol oil-portion thus obtained was subsequently rectified by steam-distillation, and its small portion, when tested for Hirschsohn's jodol reaction, yielded cineol-jodol melting at 112°. The principal cineol portion showed, after purification, the following properties : b. p. 176—177°, d_{14° 0·929, a_{D14° ±0.

It should be particularly noted that cineol occurs in *Yu-Ju* oil in considerable quantities, and the state in which the fractions up to 200° solidify by the addition of concentrated resorcin solution may be seen from the following table.

TABLE SHOWING THE RESULTS OF EXPERIMENTS FOR THE FORMATION OF CINEOL-RESORCIN.

Oil	Time of observation taken	Room temperature	Tests were executed by adding an equal volume of 50% resorcin solution to each fraction under cooling; and inoculating small crystals of cineol-resorcin, observations were taken (a) immediately and (b) after twelve hours. Temperature of distillation				Fractions		
			Up to 185°	185 to 190°	190 to 195°	195 to 200°	Temperature of distillation	Properties	%
No. 1	a	10°	+	−	−		Up to 195°	$d_{11°}$ 0·914 $\alpha_{D11°}$ +26·45°	45·0
	b	7·5°	+	−	−				
No. 2	a	11°	+	+	+	−	" 200°	$d_{12\frac{1}{3}°}$ 0·916 $\alpha_{D12\frac{1}{3}°}$ +15·65°	63·8
	b	4·5°	+	+	+	+			
No. 3	a	11°	+	÷	−		" 197°	$d_{12°}$ 0·926 $\alpha_{D12°}$ +17·70°	45·0
	b	4·5°	+	+	+				
No. 4	a	11°	+	+	−		" 195°	$d_{11°}$ 0·920 $\alpha_{D11°}$ +19·00°	33·4
	b	4·5°	+	+	+				
No. 5	a	11°	−	−	−		" 195°	$d_{8°}$ 0·915 $\alpha_{D8°}$ +25·00°	37·5
	b	4·5°	?	−	−				
No. 6	a	11°	−	−	−		" 190°	$d_{12°}$ 0·905 $\alpha_{D12°}$ +26·20°	16·5
	b	4·5°	+	+	+	·			
No. 7	a	10°	−	?	−		" 195°	$d_{13°}$ 0·911 $\alpha_{D13°}$ +28·00°	33·0
	b	7·5°	−	−	−				
No. 8	a	11°		−		−	" 190°	$d_{12°}$ 0·908 $\alpha_{D12°}$ +25·64°	23·5
	b	4·5°		+		−			
No. 9	a	11°		+	−		" 195°	$d_{12°}$ 0·921 $\alpha_{D12°}$ +22·30°	34·0
	b	4·5°		+	+				
No. 10	a	13°	+	−	−		" 195°	$d_{10°}$ 0·917 $\alpha_{D10°}$ +24·00°	37·6
	b	4·5°	+	+	?				
No. 11 (a)	a	13°		+	+	+	" 195°	$d_{12°}$ 0·918 $\alpha_{D12°}$ +17·75°	44·0
	b	7·5°		+	+	+			
No. 11 (b)	a	13°		+	+	−	" 195°	$d_{12°}$ 0·920 $\alpha_{D12°}$ +17·75°	41·0
	b	7·5°		+	+	?			
No. 12 (a)	a	13°	+	−	−		" 195°	$d_{10°}$ 0·916 $\alpha_{D10°}$ +26·95°	33·0
	b	8°	+	+	−				
No. 12 (b)	a	13°	−	−	−	−	" 200°	$d_{11°}$ 0·929 $\alpha_{D11°}$ +28·20°	30·0
	b	8°	−	−	−	−			

By redistilling those distillates, the individual fraction of which had not entered into reaction, the following satisfactory results were obtained.

			170 to 180°	180 to 185°	185 to 190°				
Distillate of No. 5 Up to 195°	a	13°	+	+	+		Up to 185°	$d_{19°}$ 0·890 $α_{D19°}$ +22·25°	42·0
	b	7·5°	+	+	+				
Distillate of No. 7 Up to 195°	a	13°	+	+	−		″ 185°	$d_{14\frac{1}{2}°}$ 0·887 $α_{D14\frac{1}{2}°}$ +24·50°	—
	b	7·5°	+	+	−				
Distillate of No. 12(b) Up to 200°	a	13°	+	+	+		″ 190°	$d_{19°}$ 0·900 $α_{D19°}$ +23·45°	60·0
	b	7·5°	+	+	+				

Thus, it will be plainly seen that the presence of cineol in all the samples of *Yu-Ju* oils, when twice distilled at ordinary pressure, can be conclusively proved by its behaviour towards resorcin.

One of the hydrocarbon fractions mentioned above, when freed as far as possible by filtration under cooling from cineol-resorcin and subsequently purified by steam-distillation, was found to possess the following constants: $d_{24°}$ 0·857, $α_{D24°}$ +3·00°. This fraction was distilled once more, and the resulting oil-portion, boiling between 175 and 176°, was submitted to the preparation of dipentene tetrabromide, according to Godlewsky's method, when, as the product, tetrabromide of the m. p. 124—125° was easily obtained. The unaltered oil-portion with the constants: $d_{25°}$ 0·891, $α_{D25°}$ +12·45°, from which cineol had not been removed, also yielded dipentene tetrabromide freely. Hence the presence of **dipentene** was confirmed.

II. The Camphor Fraction.

In addition to **camphor**, which was naturally found in this fraction, a-**terpineol** was proved to be present. When the fraction was twice fractionally distilled *in vacuo* (17—18 mm.), a fraction (b. p.

110—112° at 17 mm., $d_{11°}$ 1·027) near the boiling point of safrol began to show a lævorotary power ($a_{D11°}$ −4·15°), while the corresponding terpineol fraction had the following constants : b. p. 105—107° (18 mm.), $d_{20°}$ 0·969, $a_{D2)°}$ +20·65°. Although this lævorotary fraction consisted for the greater part of safrol, and had not yet reached the stage of purity, it freely produced a rather copious amount of a - terpineol-nitrosochloride (m. p. 113°). Subsequently its nitrolanilide (m. p. 155—156°) and phenylurethane (m. p. 113°) with a slight lævorotary power were obtained with great ease.

III. The Safrol Fraction.

Safrol occurs to a large extent in this fraction as in brown camphor oil. The oil portion of the distillate was shaken together, as a preliminary process, with 5% caustic soda liquor in order to remove phenolic substances. Then the phenol-free oil-portion thus prepared was fractionally distilled, and from the distillate, boiling between 227—235°, a considerable yield of safrol was obtained, which possessed the following properties : b. p. 233°, $d_{16°}$ 1·106, $a_{D16°}$ ±0. At the same time, **eugenol** in the form of benzoyl eugenol, m. p. 69°, was isolated from the aqueous solution of caustic soda, which had been previously separated.

Notwithstanding the fact that the attempt to detect **cadinene** by merely testing for its characteristic colour-reaction was unsuccessful, the existence of this sesquiterpene in the oil may not be altogether denied. Further researches in this direction, therefore, will be made on the acquisition of sufficient material. The **blue oil** required no further test, readily showing its own presence by the coloration imparted to the distillate boiling between 275 and 290° ; and the properties of the first distillate of blue oil were observed to be $d_{15°}$ 1·023, $a_{D15°}$ +27·50°.

With reference to the chemical constituents of *Yu-Ju* oil, there are, apart from furfurol, β - pinene, and those described in the preceeding pages, some varieties of terpenes and phenols that escaped identification ; and while they duly deserve further researches, the present studies are concluded here owing to the fact that the general composition of *Yu-Ju* oil is almost identical with that of camphor oil. As has been stated, the richness in cineol being the chief characteristic of *Yu-Ju* oil, the quantitative determination and extraction of cineol contained in the *Kōsempo* camphor oil, which is closely related to *Yu-Ju* oil, as well as in "white oils" of our preparation, should be regarded as a matter of grave importance.

[THE END.]

大正三年四月一日印刷

大正三年四月五日發行

臺灣總督府專賣局

印刷者　横濱市太田町四丁目六十二番地
　　　　大川重吉

印刷所　横濱市太田町四丁目六十二番地
　　　　合名會社大川印刷所

www.ingramcontent.com/pod-product-compliance
Lightning Source LLC
Chambersburg PA
CBHW032354280326
41935CB00008B/575